The International Library of Psychology

THE NEUROTIC
PERSONALITY

Founded by C. K. Ogden

The International Library of Psychology

ABNORMAL AND CLINICAL PSYCHOLOGY
In 19 Volumes

THE NEUROTIC
PERSONALITY

R G GORDON

First published in 1927 by
Routledge, Trench, Trubner & Co., Ltd.

Reprinted in 1999 by
Routledge
2 Park Square, Milton Park, Abingdon, Oxfordshire OX14 4RN
711 Third Avenue, New York, NY 10017
First issued in paperback 2014
Routledge is an imprint of the Taylor and Francis Group, an informa company

Transferred to Digital Printing 2005

British Library Cataloguing in Publication Data
A CIP catalogue record for this book
is available from the British Library

The Neurotic Personality
ISBN 13: 978-0-415-20926-7 (hbk)
ISBN 13: 978-0-415-75789-8 (pbk)
Abnormal and Clinical Psychology: 19 Volumes
ISBN 978-0-415-21123-9
The International Library of Psychology: 204 Volumes
ISBN 978-0-415-19132-6

CONTENTS

PREFACE

MANY books have been written on the diagnosis and treatment of the psychoneuroses in the last ten or fifteen years. For the most part, these have been at pains to advocate some special line of treatment, whether by Suggestion, Hypnotism, Psychoanalysis, Psychological analysis, Individual Psychology, Endocrine administration or other means. The result has been, that the intelligent observer, whether medical or lay is still uncertain where he should look for guidance, and whether or not the various doctrines which have been annunciated, are so mutually exclusive as the chief protagonists make out. In this country, thanks to the writings of such men as Rivers, Hart, Mitchell, Hadfield, and Brown and of M'Dougall and others in America, the views put forward have been more moderate than has sometimes been the case on the Continent, where the reaction towards the schools has been apt to be of the all or none variety.

Before we start to treat the neurotic, however, we must understand him, and try to discover why his personality differs from the normal. We must answer the questions why a patient breaks down at all, why one person breaks down in one way, and another shows a different group of symptoms, and when he has broken down, what is likely to happen to him. When we start to inquire into these problems, we begin to understand why all the advocates of the various forms of treatment may be partially right and yet suffer from limitations, so that their methods are not of universal application, and in this book I have attempted to tackle the subject from the standpoint that the physician should be familiar with all methods of treatment, and from his experience be able to judge when to use the various weapons from his armamentarium in the course of treatment.

In a previous volume in the International Library I tried to sketch out a concept of what personality is. The nature of such a concept will naturally depend on the philosophy, which is adopted in explaining the relationship of body and mind and of the personality to the universe. Since my training has been in biology and medicine, and not in philosophy, I naturally prefer a concept which will bring the psychological and physiological aspects of a personality into line with each other. Such an approach will certainly not appeal to those who favour a dualistic philosophy, and may appear to them as a travesty of the truth. None the less it is questionable if any of the current opinions represent ultimate truth and so a concept, which enables us to connect our observations in one field with those in another, has a certain pragmatic sanction, that is to say it is valuable because it works.

It is particularly in the consideration of the neurotic personality that I believe the physiological approach to be useful, for the medical study of neurosis lies midway between neurology and psychiatry in a field where the discipline of physiological thought is a useful corrective to metaphysical speculation. Much of the recent work has been done from the standpoint of pure psychology and an opportunity is given of comparing this with other concepts based on a different approach. It has been an interesting study to try to discover how far the teachings of Freud may be translated into physiological terms, for I am personally convinced that a great deal of his work is, and will come to be acknowledged, as of great service to psychology and medicine. At the same time, in common with many others, I have come to be convinced that his pansexualism is a mistake, and in the course of my own observations, while trying to keep an open mind, I have endeavoured to test this question. The results of this investigation I have tried to lay out in the following pages and at the same time I have tried to formulate some sort of survey of the ground which has to be covered, if we are to understand and treat the neurotic patient.

One of the most significant changes in medicine since the beginning of the present century is the tendency to consider the patient as a whole, instead of attaching so much importance to the particular symptoms which he may present. This results in a change in the therapeutic outlook as well, so that there is less dependence on the stock prescription as a remedy for a stock symptom, than there used to be. There is certainly no province of medicine, where the stock prescription, whether it be chemical or psychical is likely to be so useless, if not harmful, as in the psychoneuroses. For this reason I think that a criticism of the various methods of treatment is of more service than any attempt to lay down a specific therapy. A method which one physician finds successful may quite well prove useless in the hands of another, and in psychotherapy there is no short road to success ; perseverance and experience are the only means whereby skill can be achieved.

It is of some importance not only that the physician should have an understanding of the neurotic personality, but that the general public should also appreciate the meaning of the vagaries of the neurotic—this, for the sake of both the patient and the public. It is an enormous help to the neurotic to feel that he is understood, and the public might find that, if they only took a little more trouble with him, the neurotic is by no means without a considerable positive value to the community.

Perhaps some apology is needed for the term Neurotic Personality. I admit that the pathological conditions described are much better termed psychoneuroses or perhaps, as Culpin [1] has suggested, minor psychoses. However, every

[1] M. Culpin, " The Nervous Patient," London, 1924.

one knows what is meant when a neurotic is mentioned and the phrase psychoneurotic personality sounds clumsy, and minor psychotic personality absurd. Moreover, although the term neurosis may be incomplete, as a description of the pathological process involved, I firmly believe that there is a disturbance of actual nervous mechanism, and it may be no bad thing to remind the reader that, although our discourse may be in terms of mind, we must never forget what is going on in the brain.

R. G. G.

Bath, 1927.

THE NEUROTIC PERSONALITY

CHAPTER I

THE CONSTRUCTION OF A PERSONALITY

IF we are to try to gain some idea of the neurotic personality, we must first of all be clear as to what we mean by personality. Many meanings are attached to this term, and at the present moment a good deal is being written on the subject of character and personality, but it is still difficult to find any absolute agreement on the definition. As used here, the term personality includes what is meant by both ego and character. It involves all the heredity of the individual, that is, all the bodily and mental dispositions, both actual and potential, with which he is equipped at birth. It comprises the influence which race and ancestry contribute to the make-up of the individual and in this connexion it must be recognized that, although the dispositions which constitute the equipment with which each individual starts out in life may be qualitatively common to all humanity, they are not so quantitatively, and abnormalities in their relative proportion are of great importance in determining behaviour. Personality also involves all the modifications which have been impressed upon the individual from his environment. Some of these are prenatal, though relatively these are unimportant, and it is improbable that many such modifications are potent after the sixth week of intra-uterine life. The post-natal influences depend on the race, the social position of the individual, on his relations to the rest of his family, on his educational *ménage*, on the career he chooses or which is chosen for him, on marriage, on children, and on the whole gamut of his social relationship. Still, we must remember that the most striking and lasting modifications will occur in childhood and adolescence. At this time he is malleable both in body and mind, an illness may permanently affect his growth, an alarming experience may permanently modify his attitude towards a whole series of his reactions, and if he is the object of too persistent love, indifference or cruelty, his emotional attitudes may be so warped that he can never free himself from these early influences. The older he grows the more violent must be the external stimuli if they are to make a lasting impression, and as life progresses and habits of thought and action become more fixed, the more difficult is it to influence the personality for good or ill. Personality also involves all the subtle relationships between the individual and the environment in so far as his actions modify the latter. That is to say, we are concerned not only with the incoming impressions but also with the outgoing impulses of the individual, which depend not only on the organization of the personality, but also on the situation in the environment which he requires to meet. From all this is established that unity, which we recognize as personality.

In order to explain this conception of personality, we must have a clear idea as to which particular theory of the relationship of body and mind we make use of, and we must never leave out of account the unity and wholeness of personality, however much we may try to describe its structure and the manner of its building. So far as body and mind are concerned, the most useful conception would seem to be that of Spinoza, who postulated that body and mind were really identical, but presented two aspects for examination and description. One of these we study from the physical point of view and we describe its activations in terms of physiology, while the other we study from the mental point of view and describe in terms of psychology. This involves the conception of correlation, as first annunciated by Huxley [1] and modified by Lloyd Morgan.[2] As Huxley puts it, there is no psychosis without a neurosis, that is to say that every process which we describe as mental involves the activation of a certain pattern within the body. The most essential constituents of such a pattern will be the neurones of the central nervous system, but the secretions of endocrine glands and probably activations of all bodily organs will play their part. The converse will also hold good, that any activity of a pattern of structure within the body will have a mental correlate. This however is not always open to our description, since we can only describe that of which we are aware at some time or another. This means that only physical processes which have involved the highest levels of the cortex are open to the study of their psychological aspect, for although the findings of hypnosis and of psychoanalysis do throw light on mental processes which are not organized on the conscious level at the time of investigation, they must have been organized on this level at some time or another, or must be potentially capable of organization on that level, in order to be of value for investigation. However, as Lloyd Morgan has pointed out, there seems to be no reason to confine the word ' mental ' to activities at this high level and, although we cannot investigate or describe them, it is rational to suppose that some sort of mental correlate would be available for our observation at much lower levels, if we only had the means of investigating it. This is not without importance, especially in relation to the neuroses, for recent work in neurology has shown us how low-level activities in the nervous

---

[1] P. H. Huxley, *Essays.* London 1893-4.
[2] C. Lloyd Morgan, *Emergent Evolution.* London 1923.

system contribute to the complex pattern of behaviour, although their independent activity can only be observed in grossly pathological conditions, for, if structures at such low levels are damaged, behaviour is altered, although the high levels of structure are unimpaired. It is reasonable to suppose therefore, that, when we are considering a personality from the psychological aspect, some of the obscurities which have been met with in our attempts at deeper analysis depend on abnormalities in mental activity below the level at which we can hope for accurate observation. For example, the psychological influence of disease may depend not only on the consciously perceived patterns of pain and discomfort, but also on modifications at lower levels. It is probable that these low-level mental experiences have much to do with that which is called ' cœnæsthesia.' This is generally described as the sense of well-being or ill-being depending on bodily functions, but still psychologists experience great difficulty in describing its exact nature. Again, the affective states of pleasure and unpleasure admittedly depend upon functions of bodily structures under the control of the vegetative nervous system, and we can have a vague idea of what we mean by pleasure and unpleasure, but when we come to try to describe exactly what these states are, we are forced to admit that this is impossible, and that any attempt to analyse them or express them in terms of any known mental experience is beyond our powers.

If we are to understand this correlation we must investigate the formations of patterns of mental activity or of behaviour as they correspond to patterns or engrams, as Semon has called them, of structural arrangement. The engraphic patterns which represent the hereditary dispositions of bodily and mental structure present at birth are more or less definite and are recognized as the instinctive dispositions. Semon [1]

---

[1] R. Semon, *The Mneme*. London 1916.

has pointed out the importance of the permanent modification of such structural patterns by any stimulus impinging upon them, and these definite hereditary patterns are influenced in this way from birth onwards by the stimuli proceeding from the environment. Moreover, as life proceeds, the patterns may be combined and dispersed in various ways, so that new groupings occur of a more or less permanent nature. Original patterns may be very much modified in this way, although it is generally possible from the mental aspect to distinguish the influence of the definite instinctive hereditary dispositions in any given behaviour, however complicated, and as McDougall and Freud have shown, it is these hereditary instinctive dispositions which give force and direction to all our activities.

We may picture the growth of personality on the basis of increasing complexities of engrams, which become integrated and associated, in the way which Sherrington [1] has shown to be typical of the nervous system. This applies both to the individual and to the species. In the individual, to begin with, the arrangement of neurones is simple, chiefly on the basis of the reflex response. Soon, with the continual conditioning of these responses, more complicated engrams are successively formed, which have, for the mental aspect of their response, the more complicated phenomena of ideation and emotion, sentiments and beliefs, and so on, which we shall have occasion to examine at a later stage, and for their bodily aspect, various complicated muscular and glandular responses. So with the species, in the lower animal the arrangements of neurones are simple in the extreme, but with the rise in evolutionary complexity, they group themselves into more and more complex engrams, till in man, with a great increase of nervous tissue, they become extremely complicated.

[1] Sir C. Sherrington, *Integrative Action of the Nervous System.* London 1906.

As has been said already, however complex or however simple an engram may be, two manifestations present themselves for description as a result of its activation. A subjective mental activity will be experienced, and if at the conscious level, can be detected and described by introspection ; and even if below this level, it may be investigated by special methods such as hypnosis. An objective physical behaviour can also be detected by an observer, as the second aspect of the process. This difference of aspect in recording the activation of an engram is the difference between body and mind, so that, while for descriptive purposes they are different, they are manifestations of essentially the same functional process. We therefore accept the metaphysical standpoint, which makes no distinction between Body and Mind except in respect of the causal laws, by which we explain the phenomena observed, in each sphere respectively. We take as a basis of both, the activation of groups of neurones, and describe the mental phenomena which ensue, according to psychological laws, and the bodily phenomena, which may be observed, according to physiological laws.

It is not sufficient to describe the gradual increase of complexity which takes place in the evolution of the higher forms of life which eventually lead to human personality. We must enquire as to how the necessary variations take place. We believe that evolution does consist in such progressive variations, but neither the original theories of Darwin nor the modification of these by the so-called Neo-Darwinian school are quite satisfactory. Bergson's conception of creative evolution, in which the underlying spirit of progress strives towards some definite end, but regresses from time to time to deposit matter in its course, does certainly not fit in with the conceptions which we have advanced as to the inter-relations of body and mind. On the other hand the theory of emergent evolution, which was initiated by

Alexander,[1] and developed by Lloyd Morgan, offers us a theory which seems to work in accordance with our general conceptions. That any theory of evolution represents ultimate truth is unlikely, for our knowledge is still comparatively rudimentary, and hence our theories must be largely speculative and can only aim at pragmatic sanction. The doctrine of emergent evolution lays it down, that when simpler substances combine under certain relationships with the environment, the resultant substance is something unique, which enjoys a quality of its own. This proposition may be applied in both the organic and inorganic realms to matter, life and mind. As Lloyd Morgan says : " The orderly sequence of evolution historically reviewed appears to present from time to time something genuinely new. Salient examples are afforded in the advent of life, in the advent of mind and in the advent of reflective thought." [2] Modern physics has shown that all atoms consist of protons and electrons in various relationships, so that the difference between lead and gold is rather a matter of form and arrangement than of substance. Again the arrangement of atoms in the molecule makes all the difference in the emergent structure. Examples of this can be observed in the various forms exhibited by the carbon molecule, as has been shown so lucidly by Sir William Bragg. Again the various combinations of hydrogen, nitrogen, carbon and oxygen in the organic compounds show the enormous importance of form and relationship in determining variations in substances.

Before the advent of life, we can to a large extent discover and describe the exact relatedness of components and environment which is necessary to bring about the emergence of new substances. With the intervention of life, we are out of our depths and cannot discover or describe exactly the conditions under which non-living proteins can be converted into living

[1] S. Alexander, *Space, Time, and Deity*. London 1920.
[2] C. Lloyd Morgan, *Emergent Evolution*. London 1923.

protoplasm. Our present lack of knowledge, however, does not necessarily preclude the discovery of how this transformation takes place. On the other hand, it may be that conditions are such, that this relatedness was only possible at that period of the world's history when life emerged, and that such conditions can never again be repeated. When we come to consider living organisms we can trace the emergence of multicellular forms of life from unicellular forms, and, with greater or less accuracy, trace the emergence of the various species in the invertebrate and vertebrate classes.

In our present study the chief interest is centred on the growth and development of the nervous system, both in its structure and function. As has been said above, in the lower forms of life, we can recognize physiological processes, but have difficulty in describing mental processes, and in as much as we cannot determine the exact point at which mind intervenes in the course of evolution, there seems no reason to insist that something new has been introduced from without, as the dualists would have us believe.

As we now turn our attention to mental development it is not difficult to trace higher and higher integrations, but again we come to something definitely new, when we find reflective thought established in mankind. Then with the development of language and the freedom of the upper limbs from the function of locomotion and their conversion to the function of manipulation, we have potentialities of progress of which we are only just becoming aware. Nor can we foretell with any certainty to what all this is leading. Alexander [1] suggests a quality of deity, the harmony of the universe, in which all conflict, whether physical, mental or moral, shall have ceased, and the qualities of beauty, goodness and truth shall be known in their entirety. With such speculations, however, we have nothing to do at present, and our business

---

[1] S. Alexander, *Space, Time, and Deity*. London 1920.

in this volume will be to examine how certain individuals of the human race fall by the way, during their individual recapitulation of evolutionary progress.

According to Lloyd Morgan, evolution proceeds according to perfectly definite laws and according to a perfectly adapted scheme. These he describes as intervenient deity in accordance with which the evolutionary process gets itself evolved.

In the scheme of emergence we must note that the higher planes always involve the lower ; the atom cannot exist without its electrical charges nor the molecule without the atom nor the living protoplasm without its proteins. The complicated patterns of the nervous system cannot be constituted without the simple reflex arcs, and recent psychological developments have shown how the most complicated mental processes depend on primary instincts and emotional dispositions. Under certain circumstances we can trace the devolution of these syntheses. For instance, under the influence of an anæsthetic or certain drugs, the personality may disintegrate almost before our eyes, and we shall later have to study the phenomenon of regression in relation to the neuroses and shall see how under these processes the function sinks to lower levels of behaviour, representing previous stages in individual or racial evolution.

We must regard every personality as an emergent, and in virtue of its emergence, something new and distinct. Every personality is an emergent from a variety of components. These components group themselves into certain categories which present themselves for study :

1. The various organs and systems of the body, and their respective functions. In view of its integrative and controlling function, the nervous system is by far the most important of these. The other organs and systems are chiefly of significance in the study of personality, in respect of their relation

to this system, and in so far as they are modified by it and, in turn, modify its structure and function.

2. The component parts of the nervous system itself, especially the engraphic grouping of the neurones, and the response of these engrams to stimuli.

3. The mental correlates of these activations of engrams.

4. The relatedness of these mental and physical correlates with the environment, both in so far as the environment modifies them, and in so far as they modify the environment.

Further be it noted, that however similar these components may be in different personalities, their relatedness always varies, and therefore every personality is individual and is quite distinct from every other personality, just as every chemical compound is distinct from every other chemical compound. As we ascend in the evolutionary scale, the more complex is the pattern of unities in relation to each other, and the more subtle are the differences of the resultant product, even though these unities themselves are similar. Indeed, in dealing with human individuals, we might well reverse the adage and say, " Plus c'est la même chose plus ça change."

In discussing the bodily functions which go to make up the personality, our chief interest will lie with the nervous system, which integrates and controls the activity of all other systems, messages coming up the afferent nerves to the central exchange and other messages being transmitted to muscles and glands by means of the efferent nerves. Vegetative function, that is to say the means whereby the animal lives, is primarily controlled by the vegetative nervous system, which consists of two parts, the sympathetic, and the para-sympathetic, which are mutually antagonistic and, by their dual control, regulate the rhythms and activities of the various glands and unstriped muscles. The central nervous system on the other hand, presides over posture and locomotion, posture being subserved by the old motor system and locomotion by the new. Ramsay Hunt[1] has formulated the theory that these two systems are distinct in every part, the static or postural system having its centre of control and integration in the cerebellum, its messages being conveyed by special fine nerve fibres to the sarcoplasm of the muscles. The kinetic or motor system finds its centre for control and integration in the cortex, where its messages are conveyed by coarse nerve fibres to the sarcolemmæ of the muscles. He maintains, moreover, that these two separate systems may be traced to higher levels involving definite psychic manifestations, and that these can be specially manifested under certain static and kinetic disorders to be met with as hysterical symptoms.[1] There would seem to be at least a large measure of truth in this, though other observers doubt whether the present state of our knowledge warrants quite such a clear-cut division between the two systems, and believe that Hunt is simplifying the matter rather more than the facts warrant. However this may be, we may certainly recognize a hierarchy of reactions, which are built up on the basis of the simple reflex arc. Hypothetically the simplest arc consists of an afferent neurone conveying an impression from a sensory nerve ending to a central neurone, whereby that impression is transmitted to the third member of the series, the efferent neurone conveying an impulse which starts the activity of muscle or gland. Parker,[2] in his work on the elementary nervous system, has thrown a good deal of light on how the more complicated vertebrate reflex arcs are built up. In the nervous system we find that the higher levels exert control over the activity of lower levels, by the superposition of one arc upon another and, that connexions exist between the

---

[1] Ramsay Hunt, *Riv. di Pat. Nerv. e Ment.* Florence 1924, p. 1.
[2] G. Parker, *The Elementary Nervous System.* Philadelphia 1918.

various arcs represented at any level as well as with those above and below. In virtue of this system an afferent impulse is never conveyed directly across to the corresponding efferent path, but travels from an afferent channel, spreading through the more or less complicated pattern of central nervous-system neurones, until it issues again by what Sherrington has described as the common motor path, after considerable integrations and modifications have been brought about. A good deal of light has been thrown on the nature of these modifications by the work of Pawlow and his colleagues on the conditioned response. These are too familiar to need further description here, and I have discussed them at considerable length in *Personality*.[1] As the neuronic pattern through which the impulse travels becomes more complicated, certain modifications ensue. Firstly, there is delay in the response, which may be due to the passage over a greater number of synapses, where physiological experiment has shown that definite delay does occur. Secondly, there is diminution in the intensity of the response and this is true at all levels. We find many examples of this in a study of neurotic symptoms. Thirdly, the intervention of higher arcs involves control and modification of response owing to the possibility of " choice " of more engraphic motor paths, which can act together, or in antagonism, or in series. This choice is inherent in the engraphic arrangement of the neurones, and is only in any sense free at the level of reflective thought, where one process is capable of being a stimulus to the activation of a further pattern. When we come to higher levels, we find that in the processes of integration certain activities are inhibited, while others are facilitated, and though these may be reciprocal to a certain extent they are not universally so. In ordinary behaviour the action of agonist muscles is

[1] R. G. Gordon, *Personality* (Int. Lib. of Psychology). London and New York 1926.

facilitated, while that of antagonists is inhibited and, as we shall see, in the smooth working of both physical and mental activities we can trace this process at all levels. However, it sometimes happens that this arrangement of function breaks down, and both agonist and antagonist act coincidently; this involves conflict, the fundamentally important process in neurotic illness. The nature of facilitation and inhibition is little understood and need not be discussed here, but there is unquestionably a close association with the affective pair of opposites, pleasure and unpleasure. The former depends on the state of relaxation of tension chiefly in respect of unstriped muscle, whereas the latter depends on tension in corresponding structures. The work of Kempf,[1] which is discussed in Chapter XII of *Personality*, shows how important these tensions may be in relation to neurosis.

So far as the nervous system is concerned, we may sum up the bodily components of personality, as patterns of neurones arranged in greater or less complexity. Within these and between these, activation may spread with a greater or less degree of facilitation, or the passage of activation from one neurone to another may be more or less inhibited. This facilitation or inhibition will depend to a certain extent on the pleasure or unpleasure involved in the experience which results from the activity of these patterns, and further modifications result from the facilitation or inhibition so induced.

This however is not all the story, for in addition to the form and arrangement of neurone patterns we have to consider the factor of temperament, or the influence of bodily processes other than nervous, on the activation of these patterns.

It is universally recognized that the factor of temperament in the make-up of personality is of the greatest importance,

[1] E. J. Kempf, *The Autonomic Functions and the Personality* (Nerv. and Ment. Diseases Monograph Ser., No. 28).

but until recently no great advance had been made on the old humoral theories, which divided mankind into sanguine, melancholic, choleric and phlegmatic, according to the dominant humours of the body. The recent advance in the knowledge of the endocrine glands has opened up a new approach to the study of temperament, and, although other factors than these internal secretions certainly contribute to temperamental changes, they are probably the most important influences with which we have to deal. The mood of the personality certainly depends on the efficiency in function of the various vegetative organs, for it is a common observation that constipation or dyspepsia may make a great difference to a person's reaction, and this is specially the case in the neurotic, who is easily thrown off his balance by physical ailments and readily regresses to a lower or more infantile level of behaviour, when things are not going well within his body. Cœnæsthesia, or the general sense of well-being, is the emergent total of the various sensory impressions from within the body, and its exact nature is still an unsolved problem in Psychology.

When we come to deal with the secretions of the endocrine glands, we have to keep in mind that they act partly directly by their chemical effects in the blood-stream, and partly by their action on the vegetative and central nervous systems, in the same way as do such drugs as alcohol, morphia and cocaine. It is quite probable that all organs of the body liberate chemical substances of this nature, as it is a characteristic of all protoplasm to do so, but we shall probably be wise to confine our attention to these particular organs, as to whose function we know something, and leave the effects of secretions from other structures for the future to determine. Even in this restricted field however, there are considerable difficulties, because the system of endocrine glands acts as a whole, some glands functioning in harmony and others in opposition, while others again act in harmony in one respect but in opposition in another.

Before and immediately after birth, metabolism and growth are governed by the thymus gland, which becomes less and less active as age advances, the gland finally disappearing, in the majority of cases, before puberty, for the increase in function of the reproductive organs hastens the involution of the thymus. Whether this effect is due primarily to the sex glands or whether the thymus acts as a brake on the development of the latter is still uncertain. Deficiency of thymic secretions causes a weakness of the muscles, deficient calcification of bones and general metabolic upset. Over-secretion of this gland results in a hypersensitivity to foreign proteins and a risk of sudden death from respiratory failure, associated with the condition known as status lymphaticus.

The pineal body seems to exert a brake on the development of the sex organs, similar to that exerted by the thymus gland and, when it is destroyed, sexual and mental precocity are both apt to occur. It is obvious that the relation between the two functions of these two glands with the sex organs may have a good deal to do with the vexed question of infantile sexuality, but it must be confessed that at present the true facts of this relationship are absolutely unknown.

The pituitary gland exerts an important influence on skeletal growth. The gland is divided into an anterior, intermediary and posterior part, which have different functions. The presence of the anterior part is essential to life and failure of its function delays growth of the skeleton and arrests sexual development. Conversely over-function of this part promotes tissue growth, especially in the skeleton and subcutaneous tissues and excites the development of secondary sexual characters, so that this organ, unlike the preceding ones, acts in co-operation with the development of the sexual glands, but as a rule only functions when the time arrives for the latter to come to full activity.

The posterior lobe has much to do with carbo-hydrate metabolism, and insufficiency of this and possibly of the intermediate part of the gland is associated with the syndrome of Fröhlich, in which there is delay in skeletal development. The great deposit of fat and persistent failure of the development of both primary and secondary sexual features, accompanied by a childish mentality and a marked lack of initiative, are striking features of the case. Increase in the function of the gland, especially perhaps of the anterior lobe, is compatible with a good intellect and with an imaginative force, which can be controlled and brought to the service of the subject, but when the activity is too great there may be a decided loss of control, and the patient may develop delinquent tendencies, such as lying and stealing. The anterior lobe is associated with masculinity, and the masculine type of woman probably suffers from an overgrowth of anterior pituitary substances. The importance of this in the development of the neuroses is obvious, when we consider the conflicts set up between masculinity and femininity in the same individual. Decrease in function is associated with sleepiness and dullness, though there may be outbreaks of aggressiveness such as Dickens depicted in his famous fat boy.

The function of the thyroid gland is better understood than that of the rest of the endocrine organs, since its secretion is readily absorbable from the digestive tract, and consequently the effects of administration can be closely watched. This secretion exercises a profound influence over metabolism all through life. Its deficiency in the infant produces the familiar condition of cretinism, in which both mental and physical development is arrested, and at the same time changes in the skin and subcutaneous tissues are marked. Later on in life, corresponding metabolic changes occur together with a pronounced dulling of mentality and emotional expression. On the other hand over-activity of the gland leads to an increase in katabolic activity, associated with an overaction of these functions which are known to be stimulated by the sympathetic nervous system. The patient reacts excessively to all stimuli, and mentally and physically is incapable of co-ordinated effort. He is readily fatigable, displays an excessive emotionalism and a general excitability of all his mental functions. The association of hyperthyroidism with anxiety states is commonly observable, and in some cases it is difficult to determine whether the syndrome which is presented by the patient was originally initiated by a physical over-secretion of the thyroid gland or a psychical emotional disturbance. When the condition is established, there is no doubt that a vicious circle is set up and the difficulty in controlling the over-activity of the gland makes recovery from the illness an arduous and tedious process.

The parathyroids, which are more closely related to the thyroid anatomically than functionally, are essential to life and control the calcium metabolism of the body. The importance of this function in the proper maintenance of emotional and general equilibrium is a recognized fact, but insufficient knowledge of the exact influence of these glands prevents us from drawing any conclusions as to the relationship of their function with mental health.

The adrenal bodies consist of two functionally separate parts, the cortex and the medulla. If these glands are destroyed, extreme muscular weakness, low blood pressure, vomiting and increase in the pigmentation of the skin develop —a syndrome associated with the name of Addison. Mentality is as a rule unimpaired, though there may be a restlessness and want of concentration. The effects of over-secretion are little understood, but it is certain that a good supply of this particular hormone is necessary, if a personality is going

B

to be one who is well organized and ready to meet emergencies. The person with good adrenals is likely to be of an aggressive, virile type, rather like the pituitary, but over-development would seem to lead to a lack of control of emotional reactions and a tendency to excessive fear and irritability. Underdevelopment of the gland in addition to physical weaknesses may result in a submissive, feeble, effeminate type of personality.

The internal secretions of the sexual organs are largely concerned with the development of secondary sexual characteristics. The ovary seems to prevent the development of male characteristics, but the converse in respect of the testicle is not true. The extent to which these secretions have to do with the establishment of the so-called psychic maleness and femaleness is hardly worked out, but there is a certain amount of evidence to suggest that sexual abnormalities such as homosexuality may depend on abnormal proportions of glandular tissue properly belonging to the opposite sex appearing in the organism concerned.

It is obvious from the foregoing that the temperamental factor is of very great importance in relation to neurosis, but also that exact knowledge is seriously wanted. In the last few years many workers in the field of psychoneuroses have turned their attention almost exclusively to the study of endocrinology, and too often have been led to enunciate theories which have in some measure escaped from the observed facts. Much work still requires to be done along this line, and we should at present beware of either believing or expecting too much from the results of endocrine therapy.

Although we cannot trace exactly how the temperamental factors and the hierarchical arrangement of neurone patterns combine so that the emergence of higher mental function is made possible, there does not seem any inherent impossibility that more detailed knowledge in the future will allow us to trace a consecutive sequence in the process of emergence from the simple reflex response to the more complicated mental reactions, which we are accustomed to study according to the laws of psychology. Every one will be agreed that mind, as this word is generally understood, does constitute something new, when, as a dualist has put it, it comes along, but the emergence of just such new functions takes place all through the evolutionary scale, and there seems no particular reason why we should postulate a definite break at this point. Certainly when we reach this level the patterns which are involved and whose activity gives rise to mental functions are very complex, and represent the activity of the central nervous system, of the vegetative nervous system and of the endocrine organs under complicated association. It has been seen that in the activity of all three of these great systems there is a tendency for antagonistic action, which results in a balance of behaviour capable of modification in either direction, and we find all through the study of conation a series of pairs of opposites. Similarly, in affective reactions, the balance between pleasure and unpleasure is characteristic.

The lowest forms of mental activity which come up for consideration are the appetites of hunger and thirst. Even at this level we recognize the three phases of cognition, affection and conation. Certain kinesthetic impulses from unstriped muscles convey a stimulus by way of the vegetative nervous system, which, when it activates certain cortical neurones, we recognize as hunger. The affective phase is almost pure unpleasure, while these tensions are unrelieved, and pure pleasure, when the appetite is satisfied and tension is relaxed. The conative phase is the urge towards activity which will satisfy the organic need of food and drink. Opposed to this hunger appetite is a process which may be described as the act of repulsion. The cognitive phase depends on the reception of stimuli from visceral tensions of overstretched plain muscle fibre. The affective phase is one of unpleasure, which we recognize in the case of the stomach under the name of nausea, but which is familiar in the case of other hollow viscera in the desire to promote evacuation. The conative phase leads to contraction of the viscus with relaxation of the controlling sphincter and expulsion of its contents.

More complicated than this is the sex appetite, which is a combination of appetitive and expulsive dispositions. It may be pointed out, that though sex appetite is commonly regarded as pleasurable it is only the consummation that is so, and it is only at a level where anticipatory imagination is possible, that the whole process can be pleasant. In the sex appetite the appetitive and expulsive conations seem at first sight to be differentiated in accordance with sex, the conation to fill a hollow viscus being the female part, and to empty the hollow viscus, the seminal vesicles, the male part, but neither on the physical nor psychical level are sex differences so clearly differentiated in any given individual, and it is probable that tensions related to both these dispositions are present in personalities of both sexes. Unquestionably sexual tensions do influence mental activity to a very considerable extent, and Kempf has based his whole theory of neurosis on these particular visceral tensions. The study of masturbatory and other sexual phantasies in neurotics makes it quite clear that the physical aspects of the activity of these patterns cannot be lost sight of, when considering the patient's mental reactions, and, as will be pointed out in Chapter III, a full understanding of sexual function is absolutely essential, if we are going to appreciate the difficulties of the majority of neurotic patients.

At a slightly higher level we may recognize the processes of primitive fear and primitive anger, whose conations of retreat and aggression are likewise a pair of opposites. These are not experienced by individuals under ordinary circumstances, but may be clearly recognized in certain cases of neurotic regression. Panic under the influence of mass suggestion is common enough, and the process known as running amok is familiar in the neurotic behaviour of certain primitive peoples. A similar pair of opposites may be recognized in primitive passive sympathy and negativism which underlie identification and resistance, processes of the utmost importance in neurosis.

These simple mental dispositions leading up to the " instincts " have been described in almost every book on Psychology since McDougall first published his theory in his *Social Psychology*,[1] and since I have discussed them in Chapter VI of *Personality*, I do not propose to go into them fully here. We may, however, point out that neurosis essentially depends upon the disharmony in the proper integration of just these dispositions. Of these sex is doubtless the most important, but the conflict between self-abasement and self-assertion is also of the very greatest influence in determining neurotic behaviour.

In all these emotional dispositions, as McDougall has pointed out, we may distinguish a cognitive, an affective and a conative phase, which are interrelated and cannot exist except in organization with each other. The same is true of higher mental processes, although one or other of these phases may be particularly prominent. For example, what we call emotions are affective phases of processes, which have a definite conative and cognitive phase in addition. These however may be less well defined at the level of full consciousness, owing to the greater complexity of the patterns and the conditioning which may take place in their development. In this way many different stimuli may be responsible for calling out a given emotion, and there may be a great variety of modes of action which will ensue. At the level of reflective

[1] W. McDougall, *Social Psychology*. London 1917.

thought the conation may not result in muscular activity at all, but in the activation of further patterns, leading to a chain of reflective thought. These processes were the subject of study in great detail in the old days of associational psychology. Even in these, however, muscular activity is not wholly absent, as the behaviourists have pointed out, and this is of special importance in the neurosis, when these subsidiary patterns of activity, so insignificant as to escape notice under normal circumstances, may become unduly prominent. As Janet [1] has pointed out, at the higher levels more efficiency is attained, but the violence of activity is lessened. This may be exemplified by the quiet speech of the cultured thinker compared to the violent gesticulations of the mob orator. It is all too common in the neurotic to find a regression to this more violent type of behaviour.

Just as emotion involves cognition and conation, so thought involves affect and conation, and action involves cognition and affect. The most abstract thought is not unaccompanied by feeling and leads to action of some sort, while the most impulsive action is derived from some cognitive stimulus somewhere and is accompanied by quite definite feeling. If we study the more complicated emotional reactions, we find that they emerge from combinations of the simpler affective phases of the emotional dispositions. McDougall has dealt with this fully in his *Social Psychology*, and has pointed out how such complex emotions as awe are built up from simpler derivatives—self-abasement, wonder, and fear. These emotions, whether simple or compound, take their place as part of the function of a specific engram. Given one phase of these patterns we can predict the rest. If we come across anything which is dangerous to life we may be certain that we shall experience some fear and do something to get

[1] P. Janet, *La Tension Psychologique*. (*Brit. Journ. of Psych. Med. Sect.*, 1921.)

away from the point of danger, but McDougall [1] has pointed out that there are other emotional reactions, which are met with when prospective and retrospective imagination come into play. These may arise in the course of any experience. The so-called derived emotions divide themselves into a prospective group, confidence, hope, anxiety, disappointment and despair, and into a retrospective group, regret, remorse and sorrow. Surprise is another similar emotion and joy may probably be brought into this class.

Amongst the more highly organized affective processes, we must consider belief and doubt, which are of great importance in neurosis. They involve integration at the level of reflective thought and are probably confined to human experience. Doubt is not the opposite of belief, for this would be unbelief. Further, doubt is not the same as anxiety, for the latter depends on the affective correlates of tensions, resulting from alternating prospective success or failure of conations, while doubt is an analogous affective experience translated to the field of intellectual propositions. We may doubt as to the truth of Einstein's theory, but we do not feel anxious about it. Unquestionably lower-level visceral tensions may be organized in the pattern which involves doubt, just as low-level motor activities are organized in the most finely discriminated muscular action, but the highest cortical functions of judgment and reason are necessary if doubt is to exist.

Belief is an organization of pleasurable affective patterns on the plane of reflective thought, and results from the co-ordination of judgments in respect of an object or experience into a single proposition. The more perfect the co-ordination, the freer from unpleasurable tensions will the affective pattern be, and therefore the stronger the belief. When this organization takes place as the result of logical

[1] W. McDougall, *An Outline of Psychology*. London 1923.

reason, this belief is stable and not easy to shake. When this is not so, and the co-ordination has taken place at a lower level, as the result of suggestion, the belief may be apparently strong, but will be readily shaken and controverted if a more violent opposing suggestion is brought into play. These belief patterns and their stability or instability are of very great importance in the study of all personalities, but perhaps more particularly in the case of the neurotic. Too often his beliefs are the result of suggestion and not of reason, and when they come to be upset, as they may be, when he is brought face to face with new situations, he is incapable of forming new belief patterns by his own unaided effort.

When we come to study the cognitive forms of the higher mental activity, the problem of memory immediately presents itself as both difficult and important.

According to the doctrine of engraphic representation in the nervous system a pattern once laid down may be reactivated by the same or a similar stimulus. The mental aspects of such reactivations constitute images, which may be visual, auditory, kinesthetic or of other sensory variety. At lower levels, where the full cortical functions of integration are not yet fully developed, we find a reduplicative revival of these image patterns, so that the memories which are presented resemble more or less closely the original experience. At higher levels, where integration and discrimination have intervened, the differences on representation may be very considerable. Varendonck [1] has distinguished these two types of memory as reduplicative and synthetic. The pathological processes of neurosis go on at a level, where these higher functions are certainly involved, and the question as to how closely a memory revived in the course of treatment resembles the original experience is one of very considerable importance.

[1] J. Varendonck, *The Evolution of the Conscious Faculties*. London 1923.

Unquestionably both types of memory are met with, even in dreams, which by some are regarded as subcortical manifestations. The fact that synthetic images can and do occur in the course of dreaming proves conclusively that high-level cortical activity is certainly involved.

The power of discriminating and synthesizing cognitive experience is of great importance in the development of the intellectual side of personality, and the power of language has certainly advanced this ability in the human race to such an extent, that he differs from the animal more profoundly in this respect than in any other. Once the capacity for building up intellectual systems by the processes of integration and discrimination has been achieved, the use of these depends very largely on the power of paying attention to them. Attention is a complex and difficult problem, but we find that it is more easily engaged when the pattern which is occupying the field of consciousness at any moment involves one or more of the emotional dispositions or sentiments. It is easy enough to fix our attention on incidents or images in relation to our ambitions, hates, or loves, that is to say, to the well-organized and definite sentiments, but when we come to subjects related to abstract thought, where possibly only a feeble curiosity, rather remotely related to the self-regarding sentiment, is the organizing influence, the difficulty is greater, and it is here that the neurotic is apt to fail altogether. As we shall see, it is in his self-regarding sentiment that his integration falls short.

Imagination, by which we generally mean prospective imagination, whereby we can foresee the sequence of events, depends on a successive activation of engrams. The extent to which this prospective imagination is practical and in touch with probabilities depends again on the organization of the self-regarding sentiment, and we find that while the neurotic is capable of a great deal of prospective imagination, it is too often visionary and out of touch with reality. From this we see that it is in the realm of sentiment organization rather than in the higher development of cognition that the neurotic is at fault. He is perfectly capable of logic and reason, but in the formation of the systems of belief which result from these processes, there is apt to be a lack of touch with reality and of practical applicability.

In the normal individual stability of personality is reached by the organization of the various systems of belief. These should be built up in the course of the development of the higher cognitive phases of mental activity into a definite philosophy of life. The neurotic individual is incapable of this higher integration and seldom is able to reconstruct a satisfactory philosophy of life, once the conflicts to which he is subject have disturbed that which he has acquired in the course of education. It is here that one of the chief duties of the physician arises, for without a satisfactory philosophy of life peace of mind is impossible. In those cases where dissociation is a prominent feature, so-called logic-tight compartments are apt to be developed, so that impulses and ideals, which are quite incongruous, exist side by side in the patient's mind. This may go on for a time, but generally circumstances arise which break down these artificial compartments, and so the state of mental disintegration is intensified.

We have been discussing above how the integration of sentiments makes for the development of the complete personality and, as will be seen by reference to McDougall's work, these represent organizations of the lower mental processes which we have discussed. The doctrine which he puts in the forefront of his psychology is the dominance of the personality by the self-regarding sentiment, which acts as the keystone of the arch, enabling the individual to find contact both with himself and with his environment. In my opinion the close study of neurosis cannot but confirm the importance of

McDougall's contribution in this respect, for whatever may be the underlying difficulty which leads to neurotic illness, it is the failure of integration within the self-regarding sentiment, which is the characteristic mental lesion, if we may be allowed the expression, and it is to the restoration of this integration that we have to direct our therapeutic efforts. The stable personality will be the one, as I have tried to demonstrate in *Personality*, in whom a dominant, self-regarding sentiment, controlling and integrating the conative activities from which it has emerged, works in accordance with a well-defined and high-grade philosophy of life, which affords a satisfactory plan of action all through the subject's existence. This philosophy must be comprehensive and elastic, otherwise it will break down, as so often happens in the neurotic when the individual comes up against the new and the unexpected in life.

If we try to describe the neurotic personality in terms of this definition, we would say that the plan on which he is organized, that is his philosophy of life, is unsatisfactory, and his higher organization, that is his self-regarding sentiment, is incomplete.

Certain environmental factors are of considerable importance in moulding the personality, and must not be lost sight of in considering the reactions of the neurotic. As we shall see, the difficulty in the neurotic's life is to adapt himself to circumstances both within and without himself. No doubt the intrapsychic difficulties are the more important, but the extraneous difficulties must not be forgotten, for one intensifies the other.

Climatic conditions unquestionably influence the personality, and the two factors in this influence are temperature and moisture. High temperature associated with moisture gives rise to an indolent, lazy type, exemplified by the Malays. High temperature combined with dryness leads to a violent spasmodic activity, in which men are little disposed to continuous action but are capable of great efforts. Examples of such peoples are the Arabs and the Sikhs. A cold climate seems to dispose to sustained continuous activity, and if moisture is also a feature, then a certain degree of slowness is manifested. The English and the Dutch exemplify this combination. It is clear that if the neurotic personality has to live in a climate for which he is not physically suited, another situation is added to which he finds it difficult to adapt, and so this factor may contribute to his break-down.

Although race itself must be regarded as an inherent influence, and one which in these days of easy transit and mixed breeding is difficult to assess, what Mr Graham Wallas [1] has termed the social heritage is of importance to the personality. This represents the sum of the race traditions, ethical, religious, and social, which are handed down from one generation to another, and we find that the neurotic often finds difficulty in adapting himself to a new social heritage. This is the more unfortunate for him, since his trouble often consists in the fact that his own social heritage has proved inadequate.

In this chapter we have sought to enumerate, for exigencies of space prevent any attempt to do more than this, the constituents out of which the personality may be said to emerge, and we must now turn more specifically to the neurotic, investigate his peculiarities, and indicate what can be done for him.

[1] Graham Wallas, *Our Social Heritage.* London. 1921.

CHAPTER II

NEUROSIS: A FAILURE OF ADAPTATION WITHIN THE PERSONALITY

HAVING tried to define what may be regarded as the normal personality, and having pointed out that there can be no normal individual, since every one must be a different emergent, we have still to indicate what we mean by the neurotic personality.

In this connexion it is more than ever necessary to insist on the distinctiveness of the individual personality. In medicine as a whole, there has been a tendency to think in terms of disease, rather than in terms of patients, so that physicians who meet a case of pneumonia, for example, are a little apt to feel a sense of injury if it does not correspond to what pneumonia ought to be according to the textbooks. In no class of illness can this attitude be so fatal as in neurosis, for every neurotic is a different personality and a separate problem. Rules and preconceived ideas in the treatment of a neurotic patient will certainly lead the physician into difficulties, and the patient will not benefit as he should. None the less, it is possible to indicate some general principles whereby the neurotic personality may be distinguished from the normal. In my view the crucial point, which strikes one in the examination of neurotic patients, is that they are all subject to failure in the adaptation of the various parts of the personality to each other. In our view of personality this implies failure of adaptation both within the ego and between the ego and the environment. As has been pointed out, the patterns which go to make up the personality are of a definite form, derived from that of the primary emotional dispositions. Indeed all these patterns are evolved from these emotional dispositions, which McDougall has termed instincts, and it is on these patterns that the activities of the individual depend. This being so, it follows that failure of adaptation within the personality involves conflict between these dispositions or their derivatives both in relation to each other and the environment. Freud deserves the very fullest credit and universal acknowledgment for being the first to point this out, and, though some of us cannot follow him all the way in his insistence that certain specified dispositions are always involved in such conflict, it does not detract from the credit due to him for the doctrine of conflict. Freud approached the subject purely from the psychological standpoint, and, though he admitted that conflict and repression might be explicable in terms of physiology, he made no attempt to work this out. Since our conception of personality has been built up on physiological principles, it seems to be worth while to try to translate Freud's purely psychological concepts into physiological terms. Freud's [1] thesis is that the pleasure principle, that is, the conative striving of the sex impulse (libido), comes into conflict with the reality principle, consisting of restraining influences derived partly from the environment and partly from within the personality itself. As a result of this conflict, the libido is repressed, that is to say, it ceases to be able to express itself directly in consciousness, and its manifestations become unconscious. By the term 'unconscious' is meant, that the subject is unaware of the given pattern, nor can he, by voluntary effort, cause such a pattern to be revived in consciousness. Nevertheless, this pattern is capable of reactivation under special conditions,

[1] S. Freud, *Traumdeutung.* Vienna, 1900.

and, under ordinary circumstances, certain conditioned associated patterns may be activated in consciousness. These latter appear as symbolic representations, either as thought patterns or as action patterns. Such representations are either dreams, waking visions, involuntary actions (slips of the tongue, etc.) or neurotic symptoms. The repressed unconscious patterns are kept from entering consciousness by what Freud calls the censorship. This censor is itself a pattern of mental processes representing the restraining impulses, which are responsible for the repression of the conative activity (the wishes) of the forbidden impulses—according to Freud always sexual. As Lloyd Morgan has put it,[1] this conception of the good knight censor standing guard over the mouth of the dragon's cave is effective for dramatic representation, but scientifically requires exposition. The patterns which are repressed and which act as the censor are understandable on the lines laid down in the last chapter, where it was pointed out how such patterns, starting on the basis of some emotional disposition, were elaborated and integrated into the higher sentiments or complexes. Discussions have been held at some length as to the difference between the complex and the sentiment,[2] but it is doubtful if any real distinction can be drawn between them. They are both somewhat highly integrated and complicated patterns involving affective reactions. The affective groupings within such patterns are derived from one or more of the primary emotional dispositions and are in relation to an object. The only differences, which can be substantiated, are differences in the nature of the object and the degree of order and integration of emotional dispositions. The term sentiment is usually applied to a pattern, which is ordered and integrated on lines usually found in all human beings. Thus love and

[1] C. Lloyd Morgan, *Bristol Med. Chir. Journ.*, 1926, p. 107.
[2] *British Journ. of Psychology. Med. Sect.*, 1920.

hate are the stock examples of sentiments, and are patterns of definite order, varying of course from object to object, but on the whole of a predictable nature. The term complex is usually applied to a pattern whose order is less usual, and whose object is something which is partially or totally repressed and therefore unconscious. It is clear, however, that the distinction is a difficult one to draw and not of any paramount importance.

What is much more important, however, is the question of how one pattern is repressed and kept repressed or " censored." The usual explanation is, that this process involves inhibition, and that something lower in the hierarchy is controlled and prevented from expressing itself by something higher. Rivers [1] was much attracted by the problem, and sought to explain both the censor and repression on the analogy of the normal hierarchical activity of the central nervous system. He took it for granted that unconscious patterns were of a lower order than conscious patterns, and that they were inhibited and controlled as striate activity is inhibited and controlled by cortical activity, and that the censorship corresponds to this inhibition. While having great respect for the conclusions of Rivers on this point, I believe that there are certain objections to his point of view, so far as neurotic behaviour is concerned. Repression is not necessarily an abnormal function, and many of our experiences in life are repressed, or rather, to use Rivers' own terms, undergo suppression and fusion. By suppression is meant that an activity, which at one stage of evolution was useful in everyday life, has, with the march of progress, not only become useless, but has ceased to make any obvious contribution to the total behaviour of the organism. An example of this is the mass reflex in man, which is only disclosed by complete division of the spinal cord. As a result

[1] W. H. R. Rivers, *Psychology and Ethnology* (Int. Lib. of Psychology). London and New York, 1926.

of this operation, only the relatively low-level nervous structure of the lumbo-sacral cord is able to function. Any stimulus applied to the lower limb causes defensive withdrawal of the limb by action of the flexor muscles, certain vasomotor changes, sweating, and voiding of the bladder. In the healthy man there is no sign whatever of the existence of this reflex. It has been totally suppressed, but that such a defensive reaction may have been quite useful at some stage of animal evolution is obvious.

By fusion is meant that an activity, which has been useful and normal at one stage of evolution, is no longer dominant, but still contributes to the total behaviour of the organism. A good example of this is the prespinal motor system in man which, though dominated by the cortical motor system, still contributes to the tone of the muscles. This is evident from the interference with muscular tonus and resultant power of posture and locomotion, which results from lesions destroying the functional activity of this system.

Such processes can and do occur in the mental, as well as in the physical sphere, or, to put it in accordance with our plan of approach, patterns, whose chief significance is the mental aspect of their activity, may suffer suppression or fusion just as much as patterns whose chief significance is the physical aspect of their activity. Repression in Rivers' sense, which means a witting extrusion of a pattern from consciousness, seems to be in a different category, since it would appear to involve conflict, and represent the state of affairs under which neurotic symptoms arise. In the case of suppression and fusion, the result is perfect integration and absence of conflict, and the cortical function is unimpaired, while in repression there is conflict, and integration is notably imperfect. Moreover, in neurosis the cortical function is noticeably impaired. In the physical hierarchy, as studied by the organic neurologist, we may recognize what happens when

C

one or other level is cut out, as for example in motor function, spastic paralysis results when cortical function is abolished, and Parkinsonian rigidity, when striate function is abolished. In the mental sphere, such studies are still in their infancy, but, so far as we can tell, it is more in the behaviour of cases of amentia and dementia than in cases of neurosis that we can study such cutting out of levels of function, so that the conflict characteristic of neurosis does not seem to be due to a partial or complete removal of cortical control over subcortical function, *per se*. If in the development of patterns we postulate that the more complex and elaborate mental activity involves the activation of the higher cortical neurones, we can hardly deny such activity to much repressed and conflicting material, and although dreams are often extremely inco-ordinated and present such manifestations of subcortical activity as the all or none reaction, all are not of this variety, some showing the most elaborate integration and discriminative function which is much more characteristic of cortical than subcortical activity. Further, the completeness of the censorship, as postulated by Freud, is not borne out by experience in the majority of cases, and the revival of repressed material is less difficult to bring about than is sometimes implied, and less certain and constant in action than would be expected if the process of physiological inhibition which has been elucidated by the studies of Pawlow and his pupils was operative.[1]

[1] Cf. Goddard's views on the unconscious in psychoanalysis. He maintains that repression consists in the effort to think of something else, and if we " seldom or never think of an experience we are totally unconscious of it. If this is what Freud means by its being in the unconscious, it is an unfortunate use of terms. It is not in the unconscious ; we are simply unconscious of the experience, because the neurone pattern that underlies it is no longer easily activated. . . . The unconscious, as conceived by the psychoanalyst, does not exist, and consequently cannot be used to explain in the naïve way, common to their discussion, the phenomena which they describe. Every experience that has at one time aroused the activity of cortical brain cells

If we consider this work, it has been shown that inhibition is quite a definite and predictable phenomenon, obeying definite physiological laws. It is closely allied to sleep and is, in fact, a localized sleep of certain areas of the nervous system, and, if this inhibition is allowed to spread and become general, ordinary sleep will occur. Such sleep is indeed inevitable, unless the process of inhibition is prevented from spreading by counter stimuli, occurring in relation to surrounding areas of the cortex. It would seem, therefore, that in inhibition

is recorded in these same cells, and the reactivating of these same cells, in whole or in part, will at any time produce the same consciousness, either in whole or in part. Moreover, part of these neurone patterns may be recombined into new neurograms giving rise to thoughts or ideas, consciousness, which seem fully new to us because we have never made that combination before. Moreover, such new combinations may go on during sleep, either in a fragmentary way, giving rise to the well-known incongruities and fragmentariness of the dream, or on the other hand parts may fit together more logically, as when one solves in sleep a definite problem, which he was unable to work out in his waking hours, because too many irrelevant ideas came into consciousness, through association with those elements of consciousness which were important for the problem. The term " unconscious " may have justification if it can be used in the right way. It may also be useful to designate that part of the so-called unconscious which is more easily recalled as the fore-conscious or co-conscious. When the psychoanalysts will thus translate their explanations into neural terms, or terms consistent with the known facts of brain physiology, much of the objection to it and many of the difficulties now encountered will disappear, and we shall be on the road to a true science of psychoanalysis and the unconscious." H. H. Goddard : *Problems of Personality*, p. 155. (Int. Lib. of Psychology. London and New York 1925.)

Recently Freud himself has modified his ideas about the unconscious to a considerable extent. He says : " We land in endless confusion and difficulty if we cling to our former way of expressing ourselves and try, for instance, to derive neurosis from a conflict between the conscious and the unconscious. We shall have to substitute for this antithesis, another, taken from the understanding of the structural conditions of the mind, namely, the antithesis between the organized ego and what is repressed and dissociated from it." . . . " We recognize that the unconscious does not coincide with what is repressed. It is still true that all that is repressed is unconscious, but not that the whole unconscious is repressed." . . . " We must admit that the property of being unconscious begins to lose significance for us." S. Freud, *The Ego and the Id*. London 1927.

of a pattern, the neurones which subserve it are inactive, while those subserving neighbouring patterns are in a state of definite activity. Such a state of inhibition therefore implies rest for the inhibited pattern. As Adie [1] says : " In this . . . we see a vivid and beautiful illustration of the principle of economy ; for, if sleep and inhibition are the same, then the mechanism, that subserves the highest manifestations and endless adaptations of the organisms to external changes, is based upon a state of inactivity of the most precious elements of the body, the nerve cells of the cerebral cortex. Such a state of rest and sleep is the very reverse of what Freud postulates for his repressed complex, which he describes as in a state of continued activation, always striving to find expression and with the wish or conative activity forcibly restrained by the censor or opposing pattern. There seem, therefore, to be considerable difficulties in the way of accepting the view that repression and censorship correspond to the inhibitions and control in the horizontal section, so to speak, with which we are familiar in neurology. No doubt Freud's description of the conscious, the preconscious and the unconscious as levels one above the other, made the neurological analogy almost inevitable.

Let us review for a moment the characteristics of repression, and try to discover an analogy in known abnormal physiological processes, if I may be allowed the paradoxical expression.

In the typical case we find two patterns of greater or less complexity restraining each other's activity. The general reactions of the patient are more emotional than usual, that is to say, there is a tendency for activity to be diverted through vegetative patterns. The general cortical function and control is poor, and states such as over-suggestibility are consequently common.

[1] W. J. Adie, *Brain*, 1926, p. 257.

Let us take a few examples of conflict in the central nervous system. First of all, as Sherrington first pointed out, it is characteristic of normal cortical motor activity, that the principle of reciprocal innervation is maintained, that is to say that as the agonist muscles contract, the antagonist muscles relax. Now suppose a painful injury is inflicted on a limb, say the hand, the flexors and extensors of the wrist and fingers are voluntarily held in contraction, reciprocal innervation being abolished. As is described in Chapter VIII, this condition may persist for very considerable periods, as contractures, which we include here under the heading of hysteria. Doubtless as time goes on, the voluntary contraction is replaced by altered postural tone, but whether this replacement is absolute is very doubtful, and in any case, reciprocity of activity in agonists and antagonists is conspicuously absent. Effective movement is abolished, not because one or both patterns of activity are inhibited, that is have gone to sleep, but because the activities of the two cancel each other out. It frequently happens however, that a certain degree of tremor may exist, and possibly this may be accounted for by the fact that there is not complete cancelling out, though the excursion of movement is very small, since movement in one direction tends to set up a stimulus of pain, which demands activity of the opposing pattern to restore the posture of comfort. This action slightly overshoots the mark, and so the process goes on, like the buzzing of a faradic coil. Later, this may persist as a tremor which is independent of cortical control and is due to the derangement of striate, mid brain or red nuclear function, resulting from the continual flow of abnormal afferent impulses involving both muscular and common sensation. It is quite certain that, with the upsetting of the normal cortical control and of the function of reciprocal innervation, there is an interference with the vegetative functions, which are certainly represented in the mid brain and adjacent nuclei, for vascular, temperature and trophic changes, sweating, goose flesh and the like, are characteristic of these contractures, but these disappear when full cortical function is restored by re-education. The possibility of treatment of such cases by persuasion and re-education shows that the cortical function is not inhibited and asleep, but that it is rather " held up " in a state of potential though not actual activity. It may be argued that an inhibited pattern can be refacilitated by an appropriate stimulus, and that it is therefore splitting hairs to try to distinguish between inhibition and cancelling out of activity, but to my mind the latter is the more satisfactory explanation and seems to fit in more generally with observed facts. Let us now turn to an example of ordinary conflicting emotional reaction in an animal. Most people may have observed how cattle, fed in districts where chloride is deficient in the vegetation, will come for miles with great eagerness to the salt licks, provided by nature or the peasants, so that the physiological need may be satisfied. There is, in this reaction, a strong impulse to approach the salt and most obstacles will be surmounted to achieve this approach. If, however, when she arrives at the desired goal the animal finds some terrifying person or object beside the salt, her actions are extremely instructive. She is impelled to go forward by her desire for the salt, she is impelled to fly back by the terrifying object, she cannot do both and, as a matter of fact, she does neither, the two movements are cancelled out. Meanwhile she executes certain indirect movements, stamping, licking her lips, circling round, which are expressive of either or both of the cancelled movements. At the same time her respiration rate changes and her hair bristles and doubtless other vegetative changes take place. In the case of our cow, this conflict does not last long, for she probably goes off to some other rock where salt has been placed, or the greater courage of one of her kind enables her to overcome her terror, to follow her example and approach the salt. Moreover as she has presumably no reflective consciousness, the incident will not bother her again till she returns to the same place next day, when her response is so conditioned that she hesitates for a time, but, if the terrifying object is no longer there, the conditioning of the response is soon abolished.

With the human being however, it is much more possible for the cancelling process to last longer, and in course of time no doubt, just as in the case of the motor contracture, the whole process tends to sink down more and more to subcortical levels, with greater vegetative activity and less cortical control.

Further, if the patterns which are involved are large and comprehensive, the cancelling out of cortical activity on such a large scale must diminish the general cortical function, for the cortex only works locally to a limited extent, and the activity of one group of neurones depends to a large extent on its relationship to the rest. For example, experiment shows us that, even when dealing with such a clearly differentiated area as the motor cortex, stimulation of a definitely localized group of cells will produce one movement when the stimulus proceeds from above downwards, but a different movement when it proceeds from below upwards. In the motor cortex these movements, though different, are anatomically closely related, for example they are both in the hand, but in other areas of the cortex which subserve the more " psychic " functions the dependence of one pattern of neurones on the rest is certainly even more definite and complex, and therefore mutual cancellation of patterns must have far-reaching effects on cortical function. Here then, it is suggested, we have all the processes which are characteristic of neurosis and the behaviour of the neurotic patient. Normal behaviour must depend on the avoidance of this state, in which a pattern can neither dominate or be dominated by another, while the neurotic must fail in his power of integrating his patterns, since this dominance cannot take place. This question has a definite relation to the problem of higher moral behaviour, in which, as McDougall puts it, the apparently weaker impulse is enabled to overcome the apparently stronger impulse and so determine behaviour. This has been referred to in the last chapter and has been seen to be due to a close knitting of the personality as an organized whole, especially in respect of the self-regarding sentiment. It follows therefore that the neurotic is incapable of this close knitting of the personality, especially in respect of the self-regarding sentiment. This brings us to the notable point, that it is just here, within the self-regarding sentiment that the conflict of at any rate the more severe forms of neurosis lies. Freud is perfectly right in pointing out that the conflict is between the ego ideal and the ego, but, at least in my opinion, neither the ego nor the ego ideal is by any means always concerned with sex, though admittedly the conflict does often occur in the realm of sex. In the war cases it was not simply the fright of shells bursting, nor the discomfort of wet and verminous trenches, nor the tedium of being away from home, which produced the nervous breakdown ; there was always some sort of con-flict set up between the desire to escape from all these un-pleasantnesses and the feeling that to do so was not in accord-ance with the subject's ideals of himself and his duty. In peace-time cases, neither masturbation nor any other sexual irregularity of itself produces neurosis, unless there is an attrac-tion towards such practices, associated with a sense of shame or fear of their possible consequences. It should be pointed out however, that the subject may be quite unwilling to admit, even to himself, that there is any attraction in such practices. Again, a mere sense of inadequacy is insufficient to produce a neurosis, unless there is a conflicting ambition to be someone great and effective. These examples all show a lack of integration within the self-regarding sentiment, so that the patient has no clear volition to run away or, on the other hand, to stick it, nor to be content with certain disabilities which have fallen to his lot, nor really to work with all his available energies towards his desired goal, content perhaps with only a partial realization of his end. Similarly in the case of the sexual conflict, the patient is unable to bring his difficulty into the open, and approach some really competent authority to find out what really are the facts of the case. This factor of the patient being unwilling to admit certain truths about himself, which may be extended to more or less complete repression, in which case the whole situation is forgotten, involves a further consideration. When there is intense conflict and the restraining pattern is, so to speak, hard put to it to prevent the activity of the pattern, which has to be restrained, the instinctive pattern of self-preservation is brought into play in some degree, so that the intensely unpleasant affect is mitigated by a further cancellation and the ego is protected from too great and harmful unpleasure. This is normal enough in ordinary pathological processes, but in the case of repression and " censoring," the self-preservation pattern is on a high level and not at the instinctive level of flight, concealment, etc. In mankind, the possible differentiations of this self-preservation pattern are remarkable, as Rivers [1] has pointed out, and this rather obscure manifestation, whereby too great unpleasure is prevented on the level of reflective thought, is another example of the same tendency. In the process of repression and censoring therefore, we must recognize a pattern held in check and more or less cancelled out by an opposing pattern reinforced, if the conflict is severe,

[1] W. H. R. Rivers, *Instinct and the Unconscious.* Cambridge 1920.

by the pattern which subserves self-preservation acting at a higher level.[1]

It would appear therefore, that the neurotic lacks the complete integrative function which probably belongs to the fully developed cortex. It must be pointed out, however, that no one has this function developed so perfectly, that the components of every situation which is met with can be perfectly organized and integrated within the self-regarding sentiment, so that immediate decisive volition is possible in respect to it ; this is a stage in evolution to which humanity has not yet reached. Hence it follows that given a sufficiently difficult situation, anyone may behave temporarily, if not permanently, as does the neurotic. Further this integration depends on the highest possible function of the cortex and anything which depresses this will tend to render neurotic behaviour more probable. Hence, in conditions of illness, fatigue, and toxæmia, the subject has great difficulty in dealing with conflicting situations, and thus it is not uncommon to observe temporary neurosis after great mental or physical strain, or after such debilitating illnesses as influenza, typhoid fever and the like. These cases, however, do not as a rule last for more than a few weeks or months, if the subject has been fairly normal before the onset of the difficult situation, fatigue, or toxæmia. In the more severe types of neuroses, we have to reckon, not only with a difficult situation, but also

---

[1] McDougall uses the same simile in discussing the Schizophrenic, and I would like to remark, that I had written the foregoing before reading McDougall's work, not that I would hesitate to acknowledge inspiration from such an authority, but to illustrate that if investigators are thinking along similar lines, they frequently hit upon similar ideas. McDougall says : " A closer simile and perhaps a true analogy may be found in the relations of antagonistic muscle groups, for example the extensors and flexors of the elbow joint. . . . Sometimes neither system dominates, both extensors and flexors are in continued action and the limb moves very stiffly or remains locked in a semiflexed contracture—this is the condition of the Schizophrenic." W. McDougall, *Abnormal Psychology*, p. 389. London 1926.

with some degree of inherent inability to adapt to any situation. The degree to which the two factors of difficulty of situation and inability to adapt contribute to the making of a neurosis in any series of cases will vary in inverse proportion, but even in the case when the latter factor is preponderant, much can be done by discovering how life may be made easier for the patient and helping him to achieve the integration necessary to enable him to make up his mind. In the really severe cases, which Janet has described as psychasthenia,[1] a " director," as he aptly calls him, is required, and it is probable that the patient can never do without such a person, but with his help in making decisions, a patient may get on reasonably well, without being too much of a nuisance to his relatives or too much of a misery to himself. Janet's description of the inherent incapacity of the more severe neurotic—that he lacks psychological synthesis, is expressive but not explanatory, but there is no such profound mystery about the lack of development of higher cortical function in the direction of integration, for such deficiencies in the proper organization and integrative function of the central nervous system are by no means uncommon. To appreciate this, we have only to consider the achalasias, the asthmatics, the vagotonics in the vegetative field, and the people with clumsy hands and feet in the motor sphere, the muddled thinkers in the intellectual sphere, and so on.

Hereditary influences do certainly play a part in the genesis of neurosis, and stock, which is prolific in alcoholics, drug-takers, epileptics and mental defectives, is more likely to give rise to neurotics than sound stock, but we must certainly not regard all neurosis as a sign of degeneracy, for not only may the same stock produce geniuses and neurotics side by side, but genius and neurosis is all too frequently combined in the same person. In this connexion, it should be noticed,

---

[1] P. Janet, *Les Obsessions et Psychasthenie*. Paris 1889.

that we are apt to regard perfect adaptation to the environment as it is, as the highest level of function, thus laying stress on the cortical functions of integration and control, and, perhaps, not giving enough attention to discrimination. If this function of complete adaptation were really achieved, progress would be impossible, and that is why the artist and the genius, instable though they may be, are essential to society. Further, if we regard adaptation to the environment as it is, as the summit of achievement, we are presuming that the environment has reached a stabilized perfection. This is obviously untrue, and our own failures in adaptation may be the chief means of progress, inasmuch as they make for a change in the environment. By all the laws of evolution, both we and our environment are engaged on the march of progress, and the instability of the genius and the neurotic is due to their being out of step with the environment ; the former half a pace in advance, while the latter is half a pace behind. None the less, an accident is always liable to happen, whereby they change places, for this progress is not as it were, in one dimension only, but in several. Thus, even the average man may be in step in certain dimensions, but half a pace behind in one, and half a pace in front in another. It will depend therefore, on what dimension is significant for the moment, whether a person is normal, neurotic, or a genius. The influence of parental alcoholism is a very difficult question, chiefly because it is more than probable that the alcoholism in the parent is due to an inherent instability, which may be the deciding factor in influencing the child in his tendency to neurosis. Similarly parental syphilis is a very doubtful factor, provided always that no actual congenital syphilis is present in the child. For the rest, eldest, youngest and only children seem to be the most prone to develop neurosis, but this is because it is these children who frequently have difficulties in adaptation to contend with.

The eldest child at first has the advantages of the only child in his infancy in enjoying the undivided attention of his parents, more specially of his mother. He therefore is apt to be disconcerted when the next child comes along and attention is diverted from him. This is specially apt to be the case, if he is over four or five at the time of the birth of the younger brother or sister, for by this time he is quite capable of forming phantasies on his own account to explain events which seem to him inexplicable. He may therefore make up all sorts of reasons for the diversion of his mother's attention, some of which may give rise to a sense of injustice or may involve self-reproach or self-pity, all of which are fruitful sources of conflict. Later on he may develop conflict, because he is expected to assume responsibilities for which he feels himself inadequate. This is specially liable to occur in the case of the boy, if the father dies early, and in the case of the girl when the mother dies early. It must not be imagined that all eldest children develop conflicts under such circumstances, it is obvious that they do not, but these are the situations which may present most difficulty, and over which the more sensitive and inadaptable child may come to grief.

The youngest child has rather different problems to face. He suffers from the disadvantages of the only child in later childhood, which will be dealt with presently. Besides this, he occasionally develops a certain sense of inferiority because he is behind his older brothers and sisters, and they have advantages and privileges which he is denied. He may also be expected to compete with his elders in lessons and games in a way which is really impossible for him. This, however, will only obtain if there is a gap of three to seven years, a shorter gap enables him to rank sufficiently near to the next to avoid this situation and a longer gap makes him practically an only child.

The only child is a problem of some complexity and difficulty, for he certainly does have situations to face, which make for difficulties in adaptation and conflicts within his personality.   In the first place, his relations to his parents are peculiar, since their attention is concentrated on him, so far as their interests are concerned with children at all.   In many cases, when there is only one child and he is absent from home for long periods, the parental attention may be concentrated on other things, and so they lose interest in their child, who is left to the care of others.   The only child therefore may suffer from too much or too little parental regard.   In the former case this may be advantageous in early infancy, but later on it has various ill effects.   At first the parents wish the child to be too much of a companion to themselves and so he becomes too old for his years.   His interests are forced away from the games and the collecting of various commodities, proper to his years, to those of his adult relations.   Such children are often regarded as clever and wonderful.   This attitude feeds the pride and self-gratification of the parents, while it fosters priggishness and conceit in the child.   In later childhood, on the other hand, the parents wish to keep the child as a plaything and fear to lose him when he grows up, and hence tend to blind themselves to his advancing years and increasing demands, with inevitable conflict and distress.   For the child the years of adolescence when he is breaking away from the support of home and trying his wings in the world outside must be difficult in any event, but, if he is further handicapped by the attempt of the parents to curtail his further advance, it is no wonder he gets into difficulties and finds that adaptation is hard.   Another factor comes in more strongly with the only child than with others, since he is thrown more intimately into contact with the parents, and has not the diversion which other children enjoy from attachments to brothers and sisters.   This factor is the want of balance in his attachment to the two parents.   Usually the boy will prefer the mother and the girl the father, and the preference may become very pronounced, to the great detriment of the child's happiness in after life. This situation is discussed in Chapter III.

Apart from the parents, the only child is at a disadvantage as a rule because of the want of intimate attachment to children of about his own age. He may have plenty of other children to play with, go to any amount of parties and so on, but there is no one to whom he can really confide his innermost secrets, his griefs and his hardships. If he feels badly treated by his parents or elders, there is no one with whom he can talk it out and get it off his chest. Consequently he bottles up his difficulties and weaves phantasies to explain them, and these habits may lead him into mazes of mental confusion and conflict, which are hard to free him from, even in much later life. This difficulty in finding outlet for his secret fears and perplexities is especially prone to occur in relation to his sexual life, which he finds it very difficult to discuss with his elders and cannot refer to except indirectly, or in an undesirable way amongst his acquaintances and school friends. Apart from sex, however, the only child is apt to develop a sense of inferiority in respect of his general capacity, and to weave phantasies, as to what he might or ought to do, which are apt to be quite out of proportion to reality. He is inclined to take up interests which are suggested to him by perfectly well-meaning elders, which are not suitable to his age or sex, and may lead him into considerable difficulties, when he grows older and has to adapt himself to his social entourage as he finds it. Further he may develop a quite unwarranted idea of his own importance in the world. If he has been a neglected child he will feel inadequate and of too little importance, whereas if he has been a spoilt child, he has too much an opinion of himself.

The incidence of neurosis in the two sexes has been a matter of some discussion and a good deal of misrepresentation. It has been supposed that women suffer considerably more than men, but this is more apparent than real. Women are perhaps more apt to consult the ordinary doctor about the minor types of neurosis, but any large experience in dealing with such cases soon shows that men do suffer from this complaint, and often when they do, their trouble is more severe and deep-seated than is the case in the opposite sex. An important factor however does pertain, though to a less extent now than formerly. The general training of boys favours a greater adaptability than does that of girls. However, now that girls are being sent away to boarding-schools and broadening their outlook through games and other interests, this difference is becoming less marked than it was. Moreover, since more girls are fitting themselves for professions and careers, they have more opportunities for finding the right niche for themselves in life. Previously, it too often happened that the only prospects for a girl were housekeeping and marriage, and if her interests and capabilities did not lie in this direction she was only too apt to develop a conflict between what she was, and what she would have liked to have been. Apart from this, however, the woman is probably more closely bound in her emotional attachments than is the man. This applies both in her childhood and in adult life. This, of course, works both ways : if the person to whom she is drawn by inclination and duty is one and the same, she will be all the happier and more contented, but if these two influences come into conflict, then serious trouble may be in store for her, for more is certainly expected of her in her emotional life than is the case with man. We have only to consider the general attitude of parents to their daughters in respect of duties at home, compared to what is expected of the sons, and, in the marital relationships, the divorce laws, even in their lately modified form, are eloquent testimony to the same attitude of society. For these reasons it is to be expected that in ordinary life women will be more exposed to the sort of situations which are responsible for emotional conflicts than are men, but the war showed that, given the situation, men were just as susceptible to the occurrence of emotional conflict and consequent neurosis.

The age incidence of neurosis is by no means definite, but from the nature of the underlying process, it follows that any age, at which there is a special call for new adaptations, whether biological or environmental, will be favourable to the appearance of neurosis. Puberty and the menopause, when a new biological adaptation is called for, are periods at which neurosis is specially prone to develop, but late adolescence is also a frequent starting-point, for it is at this age that new responsibilities have to be undertaken, and the shelter of the home has to be left and the buffets of the outside world have to be met. But crisis may occur at any age, and if adaptation is not accomplished, neurosis will manifest itself in some form or other. The form of neurosis will largely depend on the type of personality, who is subjected to the conflict, but this is discussed in Chapter V.

The neurotic personality then, is a personality who, owing to the circumstances of life in which he finds himself, is subjected to conflict between two patterns within his self-regarding sentiment, neither of which can gain the ascendancy and suppress the other, nor can they become integrated and so fuse with one another. Consequently they more or less cancel each other out, though activity may spread through associated sub-patterns, giving rise to a symbolic representation of their conative form, or through vegetative sub-patterns, causing visceral manifestations and affective experiences of a more or less distressing type. Or, on the other hand, some part of the personality may become split off, so that it can find no contact with the rest and so becomes dissociated. So we find that the two most important processes in neurosis

D

are dissociation and repression. They are both methods of resolving or attempting to resolve conflict, and although not mutually exclusive, tend to occur in different types of personality. It is of some interest to note that all authorities do not pay equal attention to the two processes ; for example Janet has given his interest almost exclusively to dissociation, neglecting repression, while Freud concerns himself almost entirely with repression, only mentioning dissociation to pass it by without discussion.

If we may contrast anxiety and obsessional neurosis on the one hand with hysteria and dissociation syndromes on the other, it is noticeable that repression is the chief process, whereby a conflict is solved in the former, while dissociation is the process met with as a rule in the latter. As has been said, however, they are not mutually exclusive, for, as will be seen in the hysteric, the removal of dissociation will sometimes reintensify the conflict, and repression may then take place, while in the anxiety states a state of repression may give place to a dissociation. This, however, does not alter the general rule. A further general rule may be noticed,—that the anxiety states and obsessions tend to occur in the introverted type, while hysteria and dissociation syndromes tend to occur in the extraverted types. From this we may deduce that, given a conflicting situation, repression is the method of choice for the introvert and dissociation for an extravert. No one is exclusively introvert or extravert, hence dissociation and repression are not mutually exclusive, and the two processes may be observed in the same patient at different times, or repression may even occur within a dissociated system. So far as my experience goes, however, I do believe that the more introverted the patient, the more likely is repression to take place, given the necessary circumstances, and the more extraverted the patient, the more likely is dissociation to occur. This may explain the difference in interest of Janet and Freud, for the French tend to be more extraverted than the Austro-Germans.

Above it has been suggested that repression occurs when two patterns are in mutual antagonism, so that they counteract each other and, so to speak, cancel each other out. Dissociation, on the other hand, occurs when a pattern is isolated from the rest, so that no activation passes its synapses in either direction during the period of dissociation. In repression we may picture the patterns as looking towards each other in a metaphorical sense and actively in conflict, while in dissociation they are turning away from each other, leaving one in isolation. Is it too much of a flight of fancy to suppose, that this has something to do with the same process, whatever it is, which makes for introversion and extraversion, in which attitudes the interest of the patient is turned inwards and outwards respectively? This is too speculative a subject to do more than mention it, for we really do not know what determines extraversion and introversion, whether it is a matter of variation in the germplasm or, since the individual undoubtedly can slide up and down the scale of extraversion and introversion, whether it is a change in endocrine balance. In any case I do believe that, if in a given situation, which involves conflict, the attitude of the patient is introverted, repression will occur, whereas if it is extraverted, dissociation will take place.

CHAPTER III

SEX AND THE FREUDIAN THEORY OF THE NEUROSES

IT is well known that, for Freud, neurosis essentially depends on conflicts and repressions within the sexual life and, since we must admit that though not of universal application this is true in a large number of cases, in our efforts to describe the neurotic personality, we must thoroughly examine the sex reactions in life. However, we must first consider the Freudian theory of normal sexual experience.

It is unnecessary to discuss this fully, for it has been presented over and over again in the psycho-pathological literature of the last twenty or thirty years.[1]   Suffice to say, that Freud believes that sex manifestations are present in infancy ; that at about the age of four to five the libido, the impulse towards the pleasure principle (sexual gratification) becomes repressed by cultural influences (the reality principle), and during the following latency period, only manifests itself indirectly and obscurely ; that at the age of puberty the manifestations of libido again appear.   In the normal person the goal of reproduction by the process of coitus is subserved with certain modifications and accessory activities, which can only be explained in the light of revivals of infantile sexuality.   In perverts, the method of libidinous gratification, proper to certain manifestations of infantile sexuality, have persisted

[1] See especially S. Freud, *Three Contributions to the Theory of Sex*, Washington 1920 ; and *Discussion on Sexuality* (*Brit. Journ. of Psychol. Med. Sec.*, V, 161).

through the latency period, and have not, at puberty, been dominated by the genital action pattern and relegated to the subordinate position of unimportant accessories to the act of coitus. In neurotics the repression of infantile sexuality and the pleasure principle by the reality principle has not been successful and neurotic symptoms are symbolic manifestations of imperfectly repressed infantile sexuality. The evidence for this theory is given under three headings :

(1) The wealth of material derived from psychoanalysis, which by means of a special method discloses a direct connexion between neurotic symptoms and infantile sexuality, and incidentally, that the sexual abnormalities displayed by neurotics are due, either to failure of the further development of the infantile type of sexuality, or to regressions to this from a previously fully developed sexuality. Post-climacteric perversions, such as exhibitionism, are said to be evidence of regression to an infantile sexuality.

(2) The study of perversions, which is said to reveal a direct connexion with the manifestations of infantile sexuality, described by Freud as polymorphous perverse, since they exhibit all the forms of adult perversions.

(3) The observation of infantile behaviour and analysis of children, which are said to disclose quite clearly the sexual nature of many of the child's activities.

A further development of the sexual theory is the attempt to delineate certain types of character under the designations of anal erotic, urethral erotic and so on, which are said to depend on the dominance of given manifestations of infantile sexuality. The corner-stone of the Freudian theory of infantile sexuality is that all sensuous gratification in infancy is sexual. Thus Hug-Helmuth [1] states that " skin and muscle

[1] H. von Hug-Helmuth, *A Study of the Mental Life of the Child* (trans. Putnam & Stevens). Washington 1919.

eroticism must be regarded as the most primitive form of sexual feeling," and that " the infant who finds a source of pleasure in strong muscular activity always exhibits outward signs of emotion, such as increased brilliancy of the eyes, flushed cheeks, and so forth, that are well known to the adult as indications of sexual excitement." This implies that all these activities of infancy are actually sexual, as understood in the adult sense ; but not many would go so far as this. However, Freud himself says,[1] " I wish distinctly to maintain, that the sexual impulse supplies the only constant and most important source of energy in the neuroses, so that the sexual life of these patients manifests itself either exclusively, preponderantly, or partially in these symptoms. The symptoms are the sexual activities of the patient." Again : " It seems certain that the new-born child brings with it the germs of sexual feelings, which continue to develop for some time and then succumb to a progressive suppression, which is in turn broken through by the proper advances of the sexual development and which can be checked by individual idiosyncrasies." " Psychic forces develop, which later act as inhibitions on the sexual life, and narrow its direction like dams. These psychic forces are loathing, shame, and moral and æsthetic demands. We may gain the impression, that the erection of these dams in the civilized child is the work of education, but they are probably brought about at the cost of infantile sexuality itself, the influx of which has not stopped, even in the latency period—the energy of which, indeed, has been turned away either wholly or partially from sexual utilization and conducted to other aims."

Thus all the ' impulses ' which are said to determine the behaviour of the child, and later of the adult, are said to be sexual, and arguing in this way, the Freudians talk of skin

[1] S. Freud, *Three Contributions to the Theory of Sex* (Eng. tr.). Washington 1920.

eroticism, muscle eroticism, and mucous-membrane eroticism as the primary forms of sex activity. Then they recognize that certain areas of the body are established as special erogenous zones, such as the mouth, anus, genitalia, etc. These at first have equal selective activity for stimuli, and all lead to sexual activity, *i.e.*, ' sexual ' feeling and ' sexual ' action. Thus Freud,[1] speaking of sucking infants, says: " The gratification can only be attributed to the excitation of the mouth and lips ; hence we call these parts of the body erogenous zones, and the pleasure derived from sucking, sexual." Later, under ordinary circumstances, the special zones, with the exception of the genitalia, lose their potency, more or less, and so the normal erotic sensation is confined to the proper physiological system. Under special circumstances, however, the genitalia do not achieve complete predominance, but this is shared or usurped by one or more of the other erogenous zones, with the result that various perversions arise. However, it is not only on the receptive side, that infantile sex is manifested, but also on the conative side, and the infant is described as having various wishes, or sets towards muscular activity, which are of a sexual nature. These take the form of sadism, masochism, exhibitionism, prying, as well as the apparently more obviously sexual activities of embracing, cuddling, etc.

If we examine these on a physiological basis, two questions occur to us. Are all these so-called impulses sexual at all, and can we usefully talk about specific impulses in this way, without making any attempt to define what we mean by such specific impulse, and how and from where the ' driving force ' of these impulses comes ? The various forms of so-called eroticism are evidently early sensory experiences, that is to say, simple engrams are activated by simple stimuli. For

[1] S. Freud, *A General Introduction to Psychoanalysis.* New York 1920.

example, suppose an infant's skin is gently stroked, or the mucous membrane of his lips and gums is gently rubbed, a stimulus is applied which will activate certain sensory neurone paths. If the stimulus is not too violent, the activation will travel from the sensory neurones to certain vegetative neurones, with the result that glandular and smooth-muscle activities will result, which are familiar to us as expressions of pleasure, excitation, and appetition, and with these the child will experience a feeling of pleasure, etc. At the same time, striped-muscle activities are manifested, which at this age are poorly integrated and for the most part ineffectual, but which have the general tendency of bringing the child into a position to receive more of the pleasurable stimulus. There is no evidence that any specific sex pattern is activated at all. Freud admits that these manifestations may be described as ' organic pleasure,' but insists that, because similar activities are undoubtedly sexual in the adult, they must be sexual in the child. He says, however: [1] " I know too little about organic pleasure and its conditions, and shall not be at all surprised if the retrogressive character of the analysis leads us back finally to a generalized factor." Directly the stimulus passes a certain intensity it becomes unpleasant, and totally different behaviour results. Such behaviour, resulting from purely sensory stimuli is characteristic of infancy, for the engrams involved soon become more complicated and differently integrated, as do the patterns of behaviour observed. This complication of pattern will result in a relative diminution of vegetative activity, and consequently in a diminished intensity of feeling and an enhanced predominance of thought and integrated muscular activity. In consequence, this affective undifferentiated type of behaviour is not as a rule met with in the adult in response to ordinary sensory stimuli.

[1] S. Freud, *A General Introduction to Psychoanalysis.* New York 1920.

The sex pattern is relatively late in its full manifestation, and in the physical sex act there is retained in adult life something of the primary affective, poorly differentiated ' sensory ' experience, which is common in infantile life, but a similar response is met with as a result of tickling. This latter is certainly not sexual. Hug-Helmuth [1] may be correct in stating that she observed in the kicking infant, who is enjoying kinæsthetic sensation, behaviour similar to that of the adult enjoying sexual sensation ; but it is suggested that she is wrong in deducing from this that the kinæsthetic or tactile sensation of the infant is a sexual sensation ; things which are examples of the same principle are not themselves identical. The special erogenous zones, described by the Freudians, are apparently those areas of the body in which the sensory end-organs are most abundant and most specialized, but they are not inherently sexual.

As has been said, one argument on which the Freudians base their claim to the truth of their concepts is, that it affords an excellent explanation of the development of the perversions and explains many symptoms of the neuroses, and that, even in the normal adult, stimulation of the ' erogenous zones ' induces a more or less sexual experience. These contentions can, however, be adequately met by the concept of conditioning of patterns. It may well be that, as a result of hereditary or environmental influences, one or more of these patterns concerned with sensory stimuli may become associated closely with the sex pattern, and thus take on a definitely sexual association. This is normally the case with the stimulus to the mucous membrane of the mouth involved in kissing. This may go much further, the whole sex pattern being modified and altered, so that an abnormal stimulus sets it off and a perversion results. Thus suppose some sensory pattern Y

[1] H. von Hug-Helmuth, *A Study of the Mental Life of the Child.* Washington 1919.

with stimulus X and activity Z is brought into association with the sex pattern B with normal stimulus A and activity C, the two may be so conditioned that instead of two processes taking place—

only one process takes place, thus—

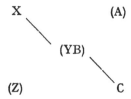

and A no longer activates any pattern, and the activity Z is no longer produced by any stimulus. This, of course, represents the extreme degree of a perversion, as for example, when ordinary sexual stimuli (A) have no effect whatever, while cruelty stimuli (X) actually produce orgasm (C), and do not in any degree produce the ordinary results (Z) ; but all intermediate processes occur, and are not uncommon.

With regard to the conative tendencies mentioned above, there seems no particular reason to describe them as essentially sexual. In fact to do so would be the result of arguing from the wrong end. No one will deny that sadism and masochism, exhibitionism, prying, and the like, as seen in adults, are associated with sex ; but the reason for this is, that the very nature of the sex act demands that the sex pattern shall incorporate certain of these patterns as part of its complex whole. The sexual act being painful on the first occasion, it is necessary that a certain degree of active cruelty and submission to cruelty should be exhibited, and in certain cases the normal sex pattern may be profoundly modified and even totally submerged by the sadistic or masochistic pattern, if these are strongly developed, thus leading to perversions, but this is simply another example of conditioning. For example, the small boy who pulls the wings off flies is not doing anything sexual, but later on his sex pattern may be conditioned by this pattern, which results in cruel behaviour, so that he becomes a sexual sadist. At first sight exhibitionism and prying seem to be more definitely sexual even in infancy, but it must be remembered that these types of behaviour are closely associated with curiosity, and that in consequence they will be concerned, not with the obvious, but with those things which custom keeps hidden. Young children will often exhibit or ' pry into ' their sexual organs, but equally often will they concern themselves with micturition or defæcation, and also with their nostrils and ears, which cannot be physiologically regarded as sexual acts ; but they have this in common, that they are all usually hidden from observation.

To sum up this argument, it would appear that the Freudians, who derive all sorts of manifestations from sexuality, are making the same mistake as those earlier critics of Darwinism, who pointed to the monkey in the zoo as their friend's great-grandfather, oblivious of the fact that Darwin postulated a common ancestry to monkey and man : so it would appear that sexual experience is only one form of primary sensory experience, and the sexual ' wish ' is only one form of primary infantile tendencies to action, all of which at this early stage of development present a considerable resemblance to each other.

The other criticism is no less important, namely, of the use of the term sexual impulse, libido, or what you will, as if it were some special force which drove on the individual to his doom. This loose use of the conception of forces is certainly responsible for the wanderings of many less erudite psychologists from the paths of probability. We have no right to postulate forces, the evidence of whose existence can only be drawn from our own imaginations, and those who seek to defend themselves behind the skirts of M. Bergson's élan vital, which many seem to do, forget that, though a concept may be valuable and justified in the realm of metaphysics, it can by no means be translated without modification into the realm of physiology. Not to put too fine a point on our criticisms, we may allow that so-called ' energy ' becomes available as the result of chemical changes, and that, when these chemical processes have achieved a certain relatedness, we encounter the phenomenon of life, and our chemical changes become biochemical changes. It is time that the ' new psychologists ' tried to explain their theories in terms of the influence of biochemical changes on afferent end-organs, neurone patterns, efferent end-organs, and muscular and glandular activities. Many psychologists will insist that this is cramping psychological enterprise, that if they are tied to physiology they can never advance at all. Unquestionably this is to a certain extent true, and the last few years have shown what enormous new fields have been opened by ' unbridled psychology ' ; but many will agree that the time has come to call a halt and try to correlate all the work that has been done with known physiological principles, for thereby we may advance the more slowly-moving science and control high-speed speculation. To the simple mind of the ancient, a polytheistic conception of the universe seemed to explain everything to perfection, but the squabbling of the Olympians reduced the old philosophers to despair. So the facile description of warring impulses, each with its own driving force, is proving a thicket of thorns, and we shall really get our ideas more clearly arranged, if we try to explain behaviour in physiological terms and confine our attention to the principles of facilitation, inhibition, and conditioning, which have been firmly established by Pawlow, Sherrington, and others.

To return once more to sex, it is suggested that in infancy there is no specialized sexual energy, since all energy must be derived from combustion of food, but there may be an engram, already laid down, whose synaptic ' passages ' have not yet been so facilitated, that there is a definite serial activation from the specific stimulus to the specific muscular and glandular activity.   Alongside this engram are numerous other engrams, some of whose synaptic passages are already facilitated.   As growth proceeds and environment influences the child, these engrams and their patterns of reaction become more complicated, more closely integrated together and conditioned in all sorts of ways, with resulting new facilitations and new inhibitions.   Amongst these develops the adult sex pattern, becoming more and more involved with others, particularly with the herd ' instinct ' and primitive sympathy, conditioning and influencing more and more of the total personality, till in adult life, it plays the important part that is universally admitted.   So, many of the patterns, originally independent, become inextricably bound up with the sex pattern, and it becomes all too easy to argue, that because they are sexual now, they always were sexual, and that sex is at the foundation of everything.

But the criticism will be advanced, What of the disclosures of psychoanalysis, which has afforded undoubted evidence of sexuality in young children ?   These apparent evidences, however, require to be most carefully and strictly examined.

Almost every one will admit that Freud was perfectly right in insisting that people in general were much too given to rationalization, and that they hid from themselves the real motives of their actions, and that this is specially true in respect of sex.   Every one who has had experience of the treatment of neurotics cannot but be convinced how frequently the symptoms are based on a conflict in the sexual life, and that this disharmony is not recognized by the patient. So much is this so, that it needs the most constant self-criticism to prevent one expecting some sexual basis, and one is apt to have a definite feeling of gratification when one finds, or thinks one finds, the sexual theme for which one has been waiting. This affective experience is due to a variety of causes, and perhaps the most important is, that we ourselves are not free from the conditioning of our sex and curiosity patterns, which results from the wholesale repression of sex in our education ; hence there is a personal gratification in discovering sexual facts about others. Experience or analysis may enable us to recognize and control this affective reaction, but none the less it is there. If, in addition to this, our reactions towards Freudian theories are of the ' all ' variety, we shall be still more inclined to welcome and lay stress on sexual interpretations. But, it may be objected, the sexual memories and dreams, etc., are produced by the patient, and the physician does nothing. Firstly, this theory that the physician does nothing is very often a rationalization. Which of us in carrying out an analysis can honestly say that we do nothing, and in no way influence the patient's train of thought ? Secondly, the patient himself is suffering from that conditioning of his sex and curiosity patterns, and enjoys that pleasurable affective experience when he can endow a memory or an experience with a sexual meaning. This pleasure is intensified by the fact that he is talking confidentially to a person who is not antagonistic to sexual phantasies as is the general public, but, on the other hand, welcomes them and encourages them. Thus, in attaching sexual meanings to memories of childhood and dreams of childhood, we have to discount these important influences, the gratification induced by the activation of the conditioned sex and curiosity patterns, both of the physician and of the patient.

Another objection may be raised here, that in some cases the patients who have been analyzed have been children from five years upwards, and that the results of analysis have still disclosed sexual experiences and phantasies.   In such cases it cannot be that the ' memory picture ' brought up in the analysis is tinged by subsequent sex-curiosity in the sense referred to above.   However, it is almost unbelievable that a child of five, or even much older, can produce a series of ' free ' associations, without being influenced to a very considerable extent by the physician.   Personally, I have not had experience of analyzing, or attempting to analyze, very young children, but I have tried to do something with older children and high-grade mental deficients, and I must confess that there was a great deal of suggestion in the result.   This does not mean, that such suggestion may not be of therapeutic benefit ; I believe that it certainly is.

One reason why memories and dreams of childhood were so easily accepted at their face value by the Freudians, is that they seem to have gone back to the old idea, that memories are stored in the mind, like bottles in a cellar, and that, in order to restore them, one went down into the cellar and brought up the bottles—a little dusty perhaps, but still the same bottles.   This concept was discarded by academic psychology years ago, and there is no reason whatever why it should be revived.   Memory is a very complex subject, and no adequate explanation is perhaps even now at our service ; but if it is reduced to its simplest terms from the physiological standpoint, we must realize that all that is retained is a conditional potentiality of restoration.   If an engram is activated by a stimulus, then it will be modified as a result of the activation and made more of a coherent entity than it was before.   If the stimulus is a powerful one, then the next time that the engram is activated, the psychical and physical behaviour (thought, feeling and muscular action)

will be more or less identical; but the pattern of reaction
is again modified as the result of this activation, and so gradually the engram, although established as a coherent whole,
is considerable altered, and before long the recalled ' memory '
differs materially from the original experience. This is what
usually happens, as may be shown by the comparison of a
recalled memory of an event and a contemporary record.
It may happen, perhaps, as a result of endocrine activities,
which accompany the feeling of unpleasure, that the synaptic
junctions of this engram are inhibited and the whole is dissociated or some opposing engram holds it repressed, so that
no further activation of just that engram takes place, until
some special stimulus occurs in the course of analysis; but
even so, it is difficult to imagine that any pattern of reaction
can persist unaltered from childhood to adult life, when we
consider the enormously complicated modifications, integrations, and disintegrations which are daily taking place.
Especially is this the case under the influence of the rapid
development and intricate conditionings of the various patterns
which make up the personality, occurring with the expansion
and establishment of the sex pattern in all its ultimate rami-
fications.

From this it is clear that, apart from the influences mentioned above, it is unlikely that a memory recalled from childhood is a true representation of past experience; but as Jung
pointed out, many of the so-called psychic traumata which
come up in the course of analysis, are nothing but phantasies
projected back into the past, if one may use such an expression.
The following case may illustrate my meaning.

A homosexual, aged twenty-nine, had an obsession for
looking at the genitalia of other men. This dated back to the
age of five. At first sight, this seemed to be obviously a case
of infantile sexuality. That the obsession and its gratification
served as a sexual stimulus now, was unquestionable, and there

was no doubt that his whole neurosis was closely bound up with his sexual difficulties of adaptation. However, I decided to try my best to avoid suggestion and to discover whether this really was a sexual manifestation. He soon began to talk freely of his sexual troubles, and experienced considerable relief from the unburdening of his soul. We then tried to trace the origins of his obsession. At first it seemed to be due to some early sexual manifestation ; but there was no conviction about this, and no resistance against talking of it. He then remembered seeing at a very early age both his father and elder brother urinating, and being intensely curious. Next he discussed with some warmth his feelings of impotence and deficiency in bodily strength, which he experienced in early childhood, and how his father was the special object of his jealousy in this respect. As a matter of fact he showed clearly that he suffered from what is usually described as an Œdipus complex ; that is to say, he was abnormally attached to his mother and disliked his father. Unquestionably this was now conditioned by sex, and indeed he had an incest dream of his mother, which filled him with intense horror ; but on carefully analyzing this, it was evident that it depended on (a) curiosity pattern ; (b) jealousy of the father on account of muscular strength, with an identification with the father ; and (c) a sexual phantasy of much more recent date and not an original experience or wish.

It is difficult to describe the analysis of a case briefly, but I would suggest that in this case the neurosis was due in large measure to conflicts of a sexual nature operating since puberty ; that into this net had been drawn the patterns representing conflicts operating before puberty, which were not in themselves sexual, the obsession with regard to the penis being as a urinating and not a sexual organ, and depending on curiosity and the will to (bodily muscular) power. I can imagine many Freudians, if they give themselves the trouble

E

of reading this, exclaiming with disgust, that of course this case and others like it depend on infantile sexuality, but that the writer's own sexual repressions prevent his acknowledging it. To this, of course, there is no answer except that there seems to be a danger, when repressions are removed, that the patterns so freed come to dominate the mind too much. For myself I wish that the factors influencing the sex pattern before puberty were more clear, for then it might be possible to do something to relieve the homosexual from his numerous difficulties in facing life, a problem which hitherto seems to have baffled even the elect.

Another criticism of the evidence of analysis which is referred to elsewhere in this book is the use of stereotyped interpretation of dreams. The best example in my experience of the danger of this was in a war case.

An ex-soldier dreamt of being very frightened by the presence of a large snake on his shoulders. A snake is a well-authenticated sexual symbol, but because this is so, it is not necessary that it should always be regarded as such in dream interpretation. The enthusiastic psychoanalyst might find some infantile sexual significance in this dream, but as a matter of fact it seemed to have reference to a terrifying experience during the war. When on guard outside a camp in the East a large snake had slithered down off a wall on to his shoulders. This dream had been persistent, but disappeared when a connexion was established with this incident. It seems unnecessary to go right back to childhood to find some sexual explanation of such a dream, when the more obvious explanation served to remove it.

Shand's [1] criticism of Freudian interpretation, as exhibiting the fallacy of inductive reasoning, does seem to be pertinent. Because psychoanalysts prove, or seem to prove, a direct

[1] *Brit. Journ. of Psych. Med. Sect., The Conception of Sexuality* (Discussion), V, p. 161.

continuance between infantile sexuality and adult behaviour in certain cases, it does not necessarily mean that this is true in all cases. Dr Glover countered this with the somewhat facile criticism, that the connexion was unconscious and therefore only could be, and moreover, would be revealed by psychoanalysis in every one. But as Dr Bernard Hart has put it, the subjection of every one to the process of psycho-analysis may be rather like putting every one through a mangle before examination. The conclusion that all human beings were two-dimensional might seem obvious, but would not be true ; so the general potency of infantile sexuality in modifying behaviour may seem obvious but need not be true.

While we are inclined to criticize the Freudian conception of sexual life and development, we cannot accept that of the man in the street, that normal heterosexual attraction suddenly appears fully developed at puberty and that anything which does not conform to this must be degenerate and abnormal. Like all other impulses sex presents three aspects for study : First of all an impression of a certain sort is received ; this calls forth on the one hand a special sort of feeling, and on the other hand a special sort of response in action. Let us illustrate this by reference to the more specific reaction to danger. The impression—one of a threat to the self—may be received through various sense organs. We may see what seems to be a danger or hear a threatening sound or feel a pain, or smell or taste something poisonous, and so on. To the untutored mind of the child or the primitive, these impressions of danger are legion, but with education they are reduced in number, and as discrimination is learnt, real dangers can be distinguished from seeming dangers. Next, with the feeling of fear in the untutored mind, we see the all-or-none reaction of panic, which overwhelms all other feelings and dominates the mind. With later development in experience and education, this feeling is also discriminated, so that more or less is felt according to the impression received. Similarly with the response in action. At first reaction may be by precipitate flight, concealment, or blind attack, none of them discriminated and not always appropriate. With more development of mind, the violence of the reaction is mitigated, and the appropriate behaviour is chosen to meet the situation.

The same change in the type and degree of reaction is met with in the sex impulse, but in view of its later development, and the delay in the possibility of its full fruition, the period at which the reactions are vague and poorly discriminated is prolonged and more open to our study, if only we can appreciate it. The impressions may be received through various sense organs, as is the case in fear, and this persists in adult life when visual, auditory, tactile, and even olfactory impressions may arouse sexual feelings. It must be remembered, however, that many of these extraneous methods of stimulating the sex pattern are the result of conditioning, and are not due to inherent lack of discrimination.

Next we must consider the feeling induced in association with the sexual impulse. This is much less definite than fear, anger, curiosity, and the like, and is less distinct from the original undifferentiated pleasure feeling. In adult life, however, it is quite a definite feeling, which we can distinguish from other forms of pleasure, such as that induced by tickling, soft friction, and the like.

Next, with regard to the overt behaviour, this cannot take place till after puberty, but at first there is a lack of differentiation in the type of behaviour, as is the case with other impulses. The essential factor of this behaviour is friction of the sensitive mucous membrane, which sets off the specific reflexes. At first it would seem immaterial, whether this is achieved by masturbation, homosexual or heterosexual practices ; later, the first two methods are in most cases suppressed, while the last may become so differentiated, that satisfaction can only be obtained by heterosexual intercourse with one individual. In this differentiation, ethical considerations have an enormous influence, but the sentimental moralist must not be misled into thinking that his precepts act as more than ancillary inhibitions on more or less undifferentiated impulses to action. Later, by means of the influences induced by these and similar considerations, the personality in general and the sex pattern in particular, may be so organized that the desired goal of monogamous chastity is reached, and a proper lasting sentiment of love is established. Masturbation must therefore be regarded as an undifferentiated way of satisfying the newly reinforced, but still undiscriminated impulse of sex, which is so insistent immediately after puberty. This practice in some form or at some time is much more widespread than many people are willing to admit, and physically it cannot be said to do more harm than ordinary sexual intercourse, so long as it is not overdone.

Psychically, however, apart from moral considerations, there are two reasons why masturbation should not be persisted in, as a means of satisfying sexual desire. The first is, that it is too easy a means of satisfying an appetite, so that the demands for low-level satisfaction may become too insistent and, outweighing all other higher considerations, come to dominate the personality. It may be like dram-drinking from the secret store in the cupboard, and be fraught by much the same result. The second is more important still. Along with the development of the sexual impulse comes much of the altruism, chivalry and desirable social qualities that we strive to foster. Although the gregarious and the parental impulses work to the same end, it is the sex impulse that gives the strongest urge towards unselfishness. This sublimation may become a biological factor in sex in human beings, and is discussed below, but, if the sex impulse obtains satisfaction from the subject himself, all the outflow, all the widening of the radius of action is prevented, it is turned back on itself, and so all this impetus to socially desirable behaviour is lost. These considerations will often help a boy to give up the habit of self-abuse, and of course moral considerations in their proper proportion are of enormous importance as well, for we must use every means to bring about the condition of monogamous chastity on which our social and religious life depends. The moralist must, however, use positive helpful arguments, and avoid all attempts to control by threats of consequences. The misery caused because a boy or a girl thinks he or she is doomed to disease or madness as a result of masturbation is unbelievable, and far from strengthening the resistance, the wretched child will often give up the struggle in despair, and become more of a slave to his habit than ever.

In the same way the homosexual practices of the young should be looked upon as delays in development, rather than as definite perversions, and it must be rare that such practices persist in after-life, when opportunity of heterosexual inter-course arrives. Indeed, on asking once, whether this practice caused much trouble in a certain school in a large town, the answer was given : " No ; why should it ? For if a boy really wants that sort of thing he can always get hold of some-one of the opposite sex." I do not suggest from this that schoolmasters should cease to regard this practice as a most serious matter. They are trustees for the welfare of the majority of their pupils, and if the individual is so impelled to find satisfaction for his sex impulse, as to interfere with another individual, he must be deterred from doing so by any and every means, fear of the most severe punishment among them. If this is unavailing, it is probably advisable to remove him from the community. Yet the doctor has to consider the individual, and it may be his part to show the wrong-doer that he is not such a decadent pervert as he may think, and that the road is still open for him to enter the rank of decent citizens, who will be a credit to themselves and their community. Great distress is sometimes experienced by the growing boy at the occurrence of nocturnal emissions, and often he is filled with the most unnecessary alarm by reading in quack literature that these signify a running to waste of his manhood, that his strength is being steadily drained away and so on. Frequently he finds that the more he determines to fight against them, the more troublesome they become. If only he could learn the truth, all conflict and consequent anxiety would be avoided. The testicles, the sexual glands of the male, are continually secreting glands, which never cease their activity, though this may be intensified by sexual stimulus from any source, whether external or from the patient's own imagination. The secretion is stored in special receptacles, instead of being allowed to drain away continually. When the tension of these receptacles reaches a certain point, the nervous connexions of the whole sexual pattern are in a state of facilitation, and this may result in the activation of the pattern in such a way as to produce a mental image. This explains the sexual dream, so often accompanying the emission, but whether this dream occurs or not, when the tension of the receptacles has reached a certain degree, their sphincters are relaxed and an emission takes place. It follows, therefore, that if no emptying of these receptacles takes place as a result of sexual intercourse or self-abuse, an emission must take place sooner or later, the interval between one and the next depending on the rate of secretion of the testicles. Since this is increased in proportion to the attention given to the sex pattern, efforts to stop emissions by concentrating attention on them, only increases them. The advice that ought to be given is, that they are not only natural but necessary, and that the only wise course to adopt is to take not the slightest notice of them.

If we are to understand neurotic behaviour, we must

understand sex fully, for, whatever we may say or think of the Freudian theory of infantile sexuality, almost all workers in psychotherapy will admit that difficulties in the sex life are the commonest single cause of failure in adaptation to life, and consequently of neurosis. To the end of understanding this matter, a fresh examination of the biological significance of sex in the human being seems desirable. Freud has stated that man alone among the animals has diverted sex from its biological function to serve his own pleasure. Doubtless this may be the case, but it is also possible that with the further complication of human development, as compared with animal development, sex has assumed a new biological function, which is not present in the lower forms of life. With the growth of his powers of intercommunication, man has become more and more of a social animal. This sociability cannot be regarded as a simple development of the gregarious instinct of certain animals, for there is much more in it than the mere herding together for purposes of mutual advantage and defence. The true " social conscience " of man involves a consideration for others and an understanding of their point of view, which has its roots, not only in gregariousness but also in the workings of the parental instinct and sex. McDougall [1] is undoubtedly right in insisting that the parental instinct should not be confused and identified with sex, yet the two are often associated and one is conditioned by the other, and still more often do they serve together as contributory agencies in the emergence of a higher quality. If we follow the development of altruism or the social conscience in the human being we must avoid a good deal of cant in the study of the child. Most people now agree that the young child is frankly self-centred and hedonistic, and that the sole guidance in his behaviour towards others is the measure of its advantage to himself, in avoiding punishment and disapproval and in gaining

[1] W. McDougall, *An Outline of Abnormal Psychology*. London 1926.

rewards or approbation. It must be realized that approbation is quite as important to the child as more tangible rewards and no doubt pure gregariousness has a great deal to do with this. The desire for approbation is specially noticeable in the school period, and there can be little doubt that the tendency is for the small boy to be a bully unless the general run of public opinion is against this. An interesting question is raised, when we come to consider the amount of altruism which is experienced and displayed in the ordinary school friendship. If we look back somewhat critically on our own boyhood friendships, we realize that we have to be very careful not to imbue them with a romantic and sentimental halo, founded more on what we would like to think that they were, from our adult point of view, than on the strict truth. Admittedly, however, altruism does find a place in such friendships, specially perhaps amongst girls, but we must realize that these friendships cannot be dissociated entirely from sex, for, as we have seen, the sex impulses in man go through a phase of indifference as to object, so that this object may as easily be homosexual as heterosexual and, since opportunity so readily presents the homosexual object, this is frequently chosen for these early attachments, in which sex doubtless plays a part. However in normal development the first occasion on which the boy or the girl really experiences true altruistic feeling, is when he or she falls in love. Now he really wishes that the pleasure and welfare of his love object shall be achieved, even at the expense of his own, and this is what, in conjunction with the parental instinct and to a certain extent gregariousness, develops with a progressive widening of radius into the social conscience. It is not meant that social conscience is love, or in any sense identical with it, but that the experience of love, and the consequent modification of the ego pattern, incident on this experience, makes the full development of the social pattern possible. It must be admitted that sex cannot be dissociated from the process of falling in love and, if this is so, then sex is essential to the full development of the social conscience, sublimated and modified though it be in the process. Inasmuch as this social conscience is essential to the full development of the human being, and is present in him alone amongst the animal kingdom, I believe that this represents a new and important biological function of sex.

It is noticeable that in those people, in whom the sex impulses remain psychically undeveloped at the masturbatory level, the ego pattern remains fixed in introversion, with the chief emotional interest centred on the self, and that their social consciousness, if developed at all, is almost entirely intellectual and arid, and lacks the emotional warmth of the more fully developed individual. This as has been said consti- tutes the real biological objection to masturbation, that it tends to introvert the individual and prevent him achieving his full social stature.

Further than this the general experience of married and unmarried people is, that it is those who have " enjoyed " full sexual experience, who are more likely to show a true " social conscience " and be more generous and understanding in respect of the behaviour of their neighbours. It must be clearly understood that social conscience, as the term is used here, has nothing to do with a desire to perform good works, which is too often exhibited by the acid old maid, without the slightest understanding or generous feeling.

It is suggested therefore, that in using sex apart from the biological aim of procreation, man is not only serving his pleasure, but also subserving a very important biological function, that of developing his social conscience and function. This view has an ethical significance, for, if there is any truth in it, we ought not to regard sex as the dreadful bogey, the Djinn which, if allowed to escape, fills the whole sky, but as a desirable and necessary factor in our development.

Needless to say, like every other impulse, sex requires control and integration within the personality, and the true development of sex is not synonymous with licence for the appetite. Nevertheless, how often is the physical act of sex in marriage approached by young people with fear and disgust, instead of with the feeling that it is going to help to raise them to their full human development as social beings, and that this, as well as the procreation of children, is one of the objects of the state of matrimony.

I do not propose to undertake any discussion of the direct result of sexual conflict in relation to neurotic symptoms, for I believe that the anxiety and allied states are due to conflict, and that hysteria is the result of suggestion acting during a state of conflict of greater or less intensity. I believe that these conflicts are very commonly, but not exclusively, sexual, and that when sexual, they have relation to the difficulties experienced by the child and adolescent, in adjusting his early desires for sexual gratification to the confused and often contradictory cultural requirements of parents and teachers, rather than to the basal Œdipus and castration conflicts insisted on by the Freudians. It is important then to examine these conceptions.

According to Freud, all, or almost all, neurotics are involved in resistances, which can be traced to the influence of this Œdipus complex. The complex gets its name from the plot of the Œdipus Tyrannus of Sophocles, in which Œdipus suffers the tragic consequences of his unwitting murder of his father and marriage with his mother. In virtue of his theory of infantile sexuality, Freud claims that the infant is jealous of his father's relations with his mother, and wishes for his death on account of an incestuous desire for his mother. The memories of these feelings are repressed, but, if the individual does not win clear and sublimate these attractions in a higher adjustment, he is likely to suffer from the symbolic effects of these same attractions, attaching them, either to the original objects, or more probably, to substitutes in the shape of other people, who have assumed the rôle of father or mother, as the case may be. Freud claims to have originally discovered this complex in his patients by his method of free association and dream analysis, and that it was forced on his attention, without his having any preconceived ideas on the subject. Be that as it may, there is no question whatever, that having established the Œdipus complex as a likely discovery in the neurotic personality, the sexual symbolization adopted by the Freudians, in their interpretation of the patient's dreams and associations has made it a certainty, and in spite of the claim for a broad use of the word sexual, the usual interpretation in the literature is in the terms of frankly physical sex, insistence being laid on the wish for actual incestuous relations. Support is supposed to be afforded for this by the various myths pointing to jealousies of the father and taboos against incestuous relationship. Freud's theory of the father of the horde and the rebellious band of brothers as being characteristic of primitive society,[1] is by no means supported by all competent anthropologists, and though incest taboos are fairly universal, this fact does not prove the necessity of a preference of the primitive for intercourse with his mother or that this should be recapitulated in the psychical history of the infant.

I am aware I am laying myself open to the criticism that I am prejudiced against the idea of finding incest wishes in infant psychology, but I believe I can honestly say I am not. I do not hold that patients are in any way responsible for the conative strivings of their emotional dispositions, in the unintegrated and consequently uncontrolled state, and if I was convinced that the first striving of sex was towards actual physical relationship with the parent of the opposite

[1] See S. Freud, *Totem and Tabu*. London 1919.

sex (the Œdipus complex is of course reversed in the case of girls) I see no reason why it should not be, but I would like to give my own experience for what it is worth. I believe that lack of balance in emotional attachment to the parents is common, especially amongst neurotics and, if pronounced, is a fruitful source of trouble in adjustment to life at a later stage. In such lack of balance the boy tends to be attracted to his mother and the girl to her father. When this is pronounced, and especially if the attachment to one parent is either repulsed by him or her, or, on the other hand, interfered with by the other, serious consequences, lasting all through life, may ensue, and the situation may be exaggerated into an unreasoning devotion to the one and antagonism and even hate of the other. The patient may further develop an incapacity to manage his emotional relations, not only with his parents, but with every one else with whom he comes in contact during life. He may have a strong impulse towards demonstrative affection, sternly held in check, but not properly and normally controlled, by a shyness and reserve, so that he is never really natural in his emotional relations with anyone, and this may lead to marked failure of adaptation and neurotic symptoms. Thus far I am prepared to admit the Œdipus complex to the full, but I have never discovered satisfactory evidence, other than that which is inevitable if stereotyped sexual interpretation of symbols is employed, of these infantile incestuous wishes of a frankly physical nature. I think that later on, the impulse to demonstrative affection may become conditioned by sex, and that the repressive impulse of pride and sensitiveness acts in such a way as to produce an intense fear of the patient's own sexuality, so that he or she becomes quite unnatural in the ordinary reactions towards sex, not only in actual life, but whenever the subject is brought up in conversation, in a book or in a play. I believe the reason for this is, that there is an unconscious dread, that if he lets himself go, there is no knowing what might happen, and more particularly what rebuffs he might encounter, similar to the rebuffs he experienced with so much distress in early life. Such patients are frequently unconsciously on the outlook for rebuffs in their affectionate reactions, just as the parvenue is always imagining social slights. They are apt to be jealous of greater attention being paid to others, and if there is a transference to their physician, they imagine that he is more interested and pays more attention to other patients, and feel hurt by this. Again they frequently do not get on at home, and find their only happiness in living away from their parents, about whom they are by no means complimentary, yet, if the parents do not seem to want them, or are indifferent to them, and especially if they die, and so leave them, the patient is heart-broken. To the ordinary observer such behaviour appears childish, illogical, and hypocritical. It is childish, but it is not illogical and hypocritical, it is simply the expression of childish emotional reactions, which have never been allowed to develop with the rest of the personality, and so still express themselves in this ambivalent dissociated way. To return to the Freudian Œdipus complex, it is often stated that the observation of sexual relations between the parents is a great stimulus to the activity of this complex. Such observations are proved to be fairly common and are certainly to be deprecated, as they stimulate a child's curiosity, and since, as a rule, the parents indignantly refuse to enlighten him, he may form all sorts of erroneous phantasies to explain it, such as cruelty inflicted on the mother, or, as in one case I came across, which was probably a later accretion, a disgust for the mother, and these may intensify an emotional balance already gravely disturbed. But, whether from this cause or any other, I have not been able to find any evidence of an infantile wish on the boy's part to have a child by his mother, or on the girl's part, an infantile wish to bear a child to her father. These seem to be regarded as an essential part of a Freudian Œdipus complex and, whatever may develop later, when sexual phantasies become tinged with real knowledge of physical processes, I do not believe they are really a part of infantile experience.

Lastly a word may be said as to the therapeutic test. The analysts claim that the " revival " of memories of the Œdipus complex in its strictly physical form has a beneficial effect. Let us consider the position. There have been brought to the level of consciousness and reflective thought, within the personality of the patient, two patterns in conflict. At this level, definite modifications of the patterns are possible, in virtue of the cortical functions of discrimination and integration. If reference is made to Chapter XV, an explanation is given there as to how suggestion acts, namely as a stimulus to a pattern already existing within the personality. Suppose now we have a pattern of uncontrolled emotional attachments to one person, or substitute for that person, and emotional repulsions to another person. Resisting this, but in no way integrated with it, or controlled by it, we have a pattern of resistance to expression of that emotional attachment. This may have been derived from the various emotional dispositions aroused by rebuffs, prohibitions, etc., which have been referred to above. These patterns have been raised to the level at which the patient realizes the undesirability of (1) but (2) is not strong enough to break up (1) and achieve the desired integration and control. Thereupon the physician, with all the authority dependent on the transference, interprets certain dreams and associations to mean incestuous or death wishes towards these involved. This acting as a suggestion, activates a pattern, which we may call the incest barrier, and this comes to be ranged beside (2) and intensifies it to such an extent that (1) is now broken up and properly integrated with the rest of the personality. Freud maintains that this incest barrier is a taboo against an individual preference for intercourse with near relations, but, as has been said, this is by no means certain. It may be a social prohibition, originating during a state of general promiscuous intercourse, to protect the race and possibly the rights of heritable property and dignities, which have already originated in quite early times.

The expression "pattern number (2) breaks up number (1)" requires modification and explanation. It is probably wrong to describe one pattern as breaking up another, it would be better to say, that the activation of one pattern at a certain level results in the breaking up of the other by a process of conditioning. Compare the behaviour of the chimpanzee described by Köhler,[1] who, reacting to the stimulus of food placed outside his cage, eventually broke a branch off a tree and used it to fish the food within his reach. Here the perceptive pattern of (branch-tree) is broken up and branch becomes part of another pattern of obtaining food. That this process of breaking up can only take place at a high level, is shown by the fact that this experiment was only carried out with great difficulty, and only successful with the more intelligent animals, and then under a strong stimulus of food, when they were really hungry.

It is suggested therefore that the Œdipus situation of emotional attachment to one parent and antagonism to the other is common, and perhaps in some degree universal and, when the imbalance of attachment to the two parents is serious, it is an important causative agency in determining maladjustment to life and so neurosis, but that the insistence on the physical incest factor depends, not on real observation, but on stereotyped interpretation of symbols. This owes its therapeutic effect to the strong suggestive stimulus to the

[1] W. Köhler, *The Mentality of Apes* (Int. Lib. of Psychol.). London and New York 1925.

opposing pattern, which enables it to break up the Œdipus pattern, so that the patient can get his emotional reactions into proper proportion and so achieve integration.

The castration complex is another very general and important complex according to the Freudians, and differs somewhat in the two sexes. In boys it constitutes a fear, whether as a result of an actual threat, or of a phantasy, that they will be deprived of the male organ. In girls it consists of a fear, that they have been deprived of this, and so robbed of the advantages of masculinity. Adler as well as Freud is inclined to accept this form of the complex. All this is said to relate to infantile sexuality and to originate during the infantile period in its definite form, so that memories revived during analysis represent actual experiences. To take the case of boys first, it is stated that cutting off the male organ is a frequent threat of nurses and others, and that this inspires great fear in the small boy. Evidence for either assertion has been entirely absent in my own experience, though the experience of one observer is worth very little. Admittedly, small boys feel great curiosity about their sex organs, but that this is in any sense a phallic symbol in the infantile stage is extremely doubtful. Later on, when conflicts over masturbation come to trouble the boy, castration ideas are not uncommon, and then there may be a regression to old curiosity patterns, which, by a process of conditioning, become linked up. Still later, when the combined pattern is reactivated in the course of analysis, a story of infantile castration fears may emerge, but, at least in my opinion, the masturbation conflicts are far more important as causal agencies in the neuroses than the rather questionable infantile castration conflicts.

In the case of girls we have a rather different situation. Unquestionably, many girls from quite an early age wish that they had been boys. This may be the result of suggestions

F

of nurses or parents, who express their disappointments that the unfortunate girl was not a boy. Again, at least until lately, boys did have a better time than girls during childhood, so that the sense of inferiority in their sex is intensified as time goes on. At the same time, there is the same intense curiosity about genital organs as in boys, and the one pattern may easily condition the other, so that an apparently early castration complex may be developed. Here again, it seems doubtful if the literal castration conflict is of much importance, as a causal agency, whereas the sense of inferiority, of thwarting and of injustice, consequent on the expressed preference of the parents for the boys of the family, or the regrets felt by herself or her parents that the unfortunate patient was not a boy, are serious influences on the personality, which are very liable to make for neurosis.

If the cure of many cases of neurosis depends on the understanding of the processes of sex and their interaction in the personality, the prevention of similar cases depends on the understanding of the regulation and control of sex in the young. There are three methods by which civilization seeks to control this unruly emotional disposition : firstly, by the conditioning of this disposition by antagonistic emotional patterns, such as fear and disgust, and its consequent repression. Secondly, by diverting the activation into other patterns of activity so that the sex pattern remains unactivated or only feebly activated ; and thirdly, by endeavouring to induce understanding and integration, so that it is controlled within high-grade sentiments.

The first method is all too common, and certainly bad, because, in the vast majority of cases, sex is too strong an impulse to be successfully repressed, and imperfect repression leads to conflict and consequent failure of adaptation. The conditioning of sex by fear or disgust may be due to actual early experiences, in which the two patterns have been simul-

taneously activated in childhood. This state of affairs is met
with from time to time in women and girls who have been
assaulted as children, but is less common than some would have
us believe. More usually it is due to the continued attitude of
parents and elders, who represent that everything associated
with sex is nasty or shameful, and that should the child persist
in thinking or acting in relation to sex, the most dire and
dreadful things will happen to him, from moral damnation
to insanity or physical disease of the worst description. Such
a state of affairs in the child's mind cannot be satisfactory,
since it is bound to lead to confusion and conflict, and frequently results in an unsuccessful effort of the child to pretend
to himself that sex does not exist in himself or others and,
when his perfectly natural sex impulses force themselves on
his notice, he is apt to swing to the opposite extreme and believe
that he is over-sexed. In any case, the sex impulse does not
develop and become integrated with the rest of the personality,
and it is apt to condition attachments to objects, which are
inadequate and no longer suitable to the age of the individual.
Common examples of this are the unavailing search by young
people for mother or father substitutes, as the case may be,
instead of proper mates, since their early emotional attachments
to parents are later conditioned by thwarted and regressed
sex feeling.

There can be no question that the third method is more
satisfactory, in which the facts of sex are faced and freely
acknowledged, the natural curiosity of the child is met as
and when it arises, not with subterfuges and evasions, but with
the truth. This does not mean that, whenever a child asks a
question about sex, a dissertation on every detail is necessary,
it is only gradually that the child requires complete enlightenment, but volumes have been written on this subject and further
discussion on reasons and methods are quite unnecessary here.
Some people, however, seem to lose sight of the fact, which

Mr. H. G. Wells [1] quite rightly points out, that full understanding and free discussion of sex does not abolish it. This impulse is still present and still insistent, but, with proper development and proper integration, it is more possible for the second method of diversion to act effectively. Under the conditions of civilization it is impossible to allow full satisfaction of the sex impulses as and when they arise, economic factors, which delay marriage and restrict families, are too insistent, so that some method for control and at least relative inhibition is necessary. With the usual national genius for arriving at the correct result from mixed and little-understood motives, the English public school tradition for games probably solves the problem fairly successfully. By the insistence on games and hard physical exercise, the bodily energies and mental interests, which might otherwise be confined within the sex pattern, are diverted to other ends, and in spite of the most glaring exceptions, it is probable that the young people of this country are less dominated by sex than those of other nationalities. There can be no question that the present younger generation is considerably more frank and less repressed than their fathers and mothers were in respect of sex, and, in spite of the groans and curses of the middle-aged on the lack of modesty and restraint in modern youth, I am prepared to assert, that the latter have a smaller proportion of their thoughts and deeds occupied with sex than had their elders. After all, unsatisfied curiosity is a potent influence on behaviour and acts as an incentive in itself, especially in young people. Lack of knowledge therefore casts a glamour over sexual experience, which may be sufficient to neutralize the impulses towards playing the game and towards decent behaviour, which would otherwise act as deterrents. A clear understanding of the actual dangers of venereal disease and the responsibilities of uncontrolled

[1] H. G. Wells, *The World of William Clissold*. London 1926.

sexual activity is of real use to the young adult, but the added exaggerations of the older method of instruction often lead to the feeling that, if once sex has conquered and led to some forbidden act, the result is so terrible that lifelong despair is the only portion of the unfortunate, and that it is no use putting up any further fight.

It is suggested then, that diversion of energy is the main necessity, but, that this is given the best chance, if the facts of sex are boldly faced and acknowledged as a necessary part of the personality, to be used and directed just like any other part. However, we cannot pretend that we have yet solved the problem of how to guide the young boy or girl through the storm and stress of adolescence, and there will still be many failures and backslidings. It is probably the one social problem that most urgently cries for solution, for on it hangs such important questions as the prevention of venereal disease and control of prostitution, and from these to the tragedies of criminology and mental defect is but a short step. Greater than all these, however, is the problem of neurosis, and, if there were never any maladjustments in the sexual life, although I do not believe that all neurosis would cease, I do believe that its incidence would be very much reduced and that we should be spared many of the more severe manifestations, which are so hard to deal with. If we cannot follow Freud all the way in his sexual theory and do not admit that because, under a rigid technique like psychoanalysis, certain results are obtained, that these results represent true psychological principles, yet we must be grateful to him not only for expounding the doctrine of conflicts and repression, which were dealt with in the last chapter, but also for insisting on the great importance of abnormalities in the sexual life in the causation of neurosis.

CHAPTER IV

OTHER CONCEPTIONS OF NEUROSIS

THE most notable psychotherapist after Freud who has worked along the lines of mental analysis, is Dr Jung of Zurich. His work on certain psychoses, notably dementia præcox, with the word-association test led him to conclusions similar to those advanced by Freud, and for a time they joined forces in the newly-founded Psychoanalytic Society. In a short time, however, Jung seceded from the Freudian school and founded his own clinic at Zürich, which has attracted many well-known psychotherapists from this country to study his methods. He came to disagree with Freud on several points, notably in his conception of the libido. As has been said, for Freud this was the urge of sex, while for Jung it was the urge of life, which drove on the individual, to find adaptation and satisfaction in his surroundings.[1] Difficulties therefore lay in the present and in the future, rather than in the past, and conflicts did not depend so much on repressions of the sex impulse in the course of childhood as in the conflicting influences of the various tendencies and functions within the personality at the time of the illness.

Jung's conception of the personality is exceedingly complex, for, following Freud in the division of mental activity into conscious and unconscious, he enlarges the scope of the unconscious to a very great extent. He, as an introvert, is

[1] C. Jung, *Collected Papers on Analytical Psychology*. London 1917. Also his *Psychology of the Unconscious*. London 1916.

interested in what the individual contributes in virtue of his own inherent disposition, and therefore studies the pattern activated by the stimulus, rather than the stimulus which activates it. Accepting the Lamarckian doctrine of the inheritance of acquired characters, he maintains that many of these patterns represent "archetypes," or inherited ancestral experiences, which have never been conscious within the individual experience, yet may condition behaviour in so far as they are activated by chance stimuli.

Thus Jung would divide the unconscious content of the mind, *i.e.*, the collection of patterns not enjoying consciousness at any moment, into two divisions. Firstly, a personal unconscious, including that which has been forgotten and repressed, and that which represents subliminal impressions —in other words, all those patterns resulting from the interaction of the disposition with the environment, which have failed to reach, or ceased to enjoy, that relatedness which involves consciousness. Secondly, he describes the collective unconscious, whose contents do not originate in personal acquisitions, but in the inherent potentiality of psychic function, which is subserved by the inherited brain structure. This collective unconscious material consists of the mythological primordial images—those motives and images handed down from long-distant ancestors which apparently can spring anew in every age and clime, without historic tradition or personal migration. There are many examples, especially in the history of symbols, which seem to bear this out ; for example, the universality of the serpent and fish symbols for fertility, and the attitude of primitives to the four elementals, earth, air, fire and water. The archetypes however which Jung claims to have discovered are much more complex than these. The instances which have been given may serve to show that in the absence of obvious common environmental influences, similar behaviour patterns emerge, as if from a common source. Just as conscious content is integrated and combined to produce behaviour in the form of conscious actions and thought, so unconscious content is integrated and combined on a different level of relatedness, to produce overt behaviour in the form of unconscious actions and thought processes, such as appear in dreams or phantasies. This does not imply that any content, which at times enjoys the special relatedness which involves consciousness, takes no part in such actions and dreams ; but rather, that their set and pattern depend chiefly on that content, which does not enjoy such relatedness, and so is unconscious. This, of course, refers to activities and thoughts, which Jung would place in that division of unconscious mental activity which he calls the collective unconscious, for most of the content of the individual unconscious mind has, at one time or another, enjoyed the relatedness which involves consciousness.

Jung further regards the unconscious content as compensatory ; that is to say, when there is a deficiency in the stream of proper conscious content, so that the subject cannot deal adequately with a situation, this deficiency is made up by unconscious content. But, inasmuch as this latter content has failed to achieve that higher relatedness which we call consciousness, its adaptation to environment is primitive and incomplete, and therefore more or less unsatisfactory. It follows from this that the more one-sided is the conscious content, the more obviously compensatory will be the unconscious content, a factor which will be noticed further when dealing with the dissociation syndromes, and conscious and unconscious behaviour will be complementary to each other. Thus, in relation to the types of introvert and extravert to be discussed in the next chapter, if an individual is a marked extravert in his conscious behaviour, his unconscious behaviour will tend to be of the introverted type, and vice versa. Similarly, a person may have developed his intellectual side, but not his intuitive side, in which case his intuition is inadequate. His phantasies, dreams and neurotic symptoms however will tend to be intuitive and singularly deficient in rational control, and just for this reason essentially inadequate. Jung interprets dreams along these lines, that is to say, that the various elements of the dream are representatives of inherited racial patterns, or of undeveloped functions in the personality, and that their relationship in the dream throws light not on past psychic traumata, but on present problems which the subject is called upon to face, though failing to do so to a greater or less extent. When this failure is serious, then neurosis develops and the failure may take place, either because there is conflict with the environment, or more often, because the conflict is endopsychic, that is to say, that two or more patterns within the personality find themselves in opposition. When this occurs, the libido, unable to find expression through the proper channels on a higher level, regresses and finds outlet through channels on a lower level, giving expression to various unconscious archetypes and symbolic manifestations, which appear as the various symptoms of the neuroses. This conception of neurosis fits in with that which we have advanced, if we use the conception of various patterns activated at different levels, rather than that of the channels at which the libido finds egress, but the criticisms which we are led to advance are the multiplication of possible patterns laid down in the disposition of the individual and the meaning attached to these patterns and their manifestations. The fact of the existence of such patterns is not difficult to accept.

We have admitted Semon's theory of the Mneme [1]—the engraphic effect of stimuli, as a useful concept, which seems to explain the facts and is, moreover, reasonably likely to

[1] R. Semon, *The Mneme.* London 1916.

approximate to the truth. This theory allows for the transmission of just such characters as Jung suggests. An engram is an arrangement of neurones, conditioned in such a way that their subsequent activation produces a pattern of behaviour which resembles, but is not identical with the behaviour resulting from their previous activation. Such engrams are evolved out of inherited dispositions, by the modification necessitated by the environment. It would seem that, in this process of the evolution of engrams, two factors must be taken into account, environment and inheritance. The neural patterns or engrams are not formed simply by an imprint induced by the environment on a malleable material, as a crest is imprinted on soft wax by a signet-ring, but there is in that relatedness, which involves life, a tendency to achieve adaptation ; and so, in respect of this, an engram will take on a certain form which subserves greater adaptability in virtue of its inherent nature. In other words, it is not only a function of the environment, but also of that relatedness which involves life. This concept does not involve any special vital energy, but simply that the relatedness follows certain laws, and these laws imply behaviour which, if followed, will lead to adaptation rather than away from it. Recent experiments have shown that such engrams which are determined in the nervous system, and which become progressively adaptive in the individual animal, by some modification of the germ cell are represented in the next generation, not in their original form, but in their later form of greater adaptability. Thus, it has been found that not only will an individual animal, learning by experience, require fewer and fewer trials and errors in finding its way out of a maze, but its offspring will learn more quickly than did the parent, and the diminution of trials and errors, necessary in the learning process, will be transmitted through several generations. If this be so, then it may be admitted that engrams representing primitive patterns of thought and feeling, acquired during the life-time of various individuals, may be transmitted in their modified form to future generations.

On the analogy of motor activity, it is to be expected that such primitive patterns, which are transmitted, will be unconscious and not conscious. We must, however, be careful to keep our speculations with regard to these unconscious patterns within bounds, and to be certain that we have evidence to support our conclusions as to the meaning of dream symbols and neurotic manifestations. As is the case in the Freudian interpretation of neurosis, so with the Jungian interpretation, symbols may become too stereotyped and systematized. Thus the behaviour of the neurotic patient is held to be symbolic of sexual strivings on the one hand, or of strivings towards adaptation depending on race memories on the other, whereas in many cases the real trouble is not so very hard to discover, if we are not hidebound by preconceived notions as to what the symptom ought to mean.

Adler was the first of Freud's followers to break from the original school. He agreed that the causes of neurosis must be looked for in the mental reactions of the patient, and that the finding and reviving the contents of the lacunæ of memory in ordinary conscious life were the means whereby the genesis of the neurosis could be discovered and understood. He considers that his investigations show that the actual cause of neurotic disease is the mood residue dating from childhood, which depends on single or repeated failures in any human endeavour. Moreover he states : " Regularly and inexorably was it forced upon my attention that the possession of inherited inferior organs, organic systems and glands with internal secretions created a situation in the early stages of a child's development, whereby a normal feeling of weakness and helplessness had been enormously intensified and had grown into a deeply felt sense of inferiority."[1] This in turn leads to " a desire to possess, eat, hear, see and know everything." Such children wish to surpass all others and accomplish everything alone. Their phantasy plays with all kinds of greatness. The child's personality displays a mixture of passive and active characteristics, a feminine obedience alternating and conflicting with a masculine defiance, so that there is always an impulse to achieve complete power and independence (masculinity), but the sense of inferiority, the inherent sense of weakness, (femininity) prevents a direct attack on this goal. The individual therefore seeks to arrive at the position of power and dominance, which he desires, by indirect means, even through a display of weakness and illness. Mr Lytton Strachey, if he is historically correct, has shown us how two very notable women—Queen Victoria and Florence Nightingale—did wield their great power, very largely because they kept themselves in seclusion, one through a long period of sentimental mourning and the other through (neurotic ?) illness. So the neurotic strives to gain and often succeeds in gaining his wishes by means of his illness. This accounts for his frequent unwillingness to give up the illness, while his doubts, fears and compulsions are all expressions of his striving to attain his end. These strivings are never complete, lest he run the risk of losing the power he has gained and sinking into a state of dependency, from which he is constantly striving to escape. The goal which he seeks, and the means whereby he is striving to reach that goal, are by no means clear to the individual, indeed they may be quite unconscious, for frequently they are quite illogical and completely at variance with the circumstances in which the patient finds himself. It is the physician's task to make these things

---

[1] A. Adler, *Individual Psychology* (Int. Lib. of Psychol.). London and New York 1924. See also his *The Neurotic Constitution*. London 1904; and *Study of Organ Inferiority and its Psychical Compensation*. New York 1917.

clear to the patient and induce him to give up a goal which is impossible of achievement, and content himself with the position which is possible for him. Adler admits that sex often comes into the conflicts of neurotics, but he does not, like Freud, consider that it is the sex impulse, the libido, which drives on the patient to seek satisfaction by its *vis a tergo*, but rather that the patient is led through his devious paths towards the goal of complete masculinity. Sex then is rather an accidental complication, which may colour the ambitions and phantasies of the neurotic, but has no dynamic influence in shaping his real ends.

There can be no doubt at all that this conception of Adler's does apply to neuroses and is extremely useful in the treatment of certain cases, but it cannot be applied to all, any more than Freud's sexual theory or Jung's theory of endopsychic compensations can be applied to all.

It would be an interesting experiment, if we had before us a moderately severe case of neurosis and could triplicate him, to treat his first replica on strictly Freudian lines, his second on strictly Jungian lines and his third on Adlerian lines. As a matter of fact, if we set out to do this for the purpose of determining the relative advantage of the three methods, I venture to suggest we should not get very much further. Even though in our hypothetical case, the factors of patient and physician are constants, all three methods cannot be equally favoured by the physician, since his choice must depend to a certain extent on his own personality. Further, so complex is the personality of the patient, that it is probable, if his sex impulse and its strivings are investigated, that conflicts will be discovered whose resolution will be of benefit. Similarly, there will be conflicts between two or more functions—say intuition and sensation, and there will be a sense of inferiority with a compensatory will to power, the straightening out and reproportioning of which conflicting patterns will bring relief to the patient. As has been said, the individual patient is a definite problem, which must be dealt with as a separate field of enquiry and not be expected to fit into any special scheme. Hence we ought to be prepared to find that every worker in the field of psychotherapy has something to contribute to the general state of knowledge.

It is interesting to turn from the psychoanalytic expositions of the neuroses, to that of Professor Janet, who has worked out a theory of neurotic illness, which is singularly complete, if we could only accept the premises on which he bases his arguments. He believes that neurosis depends on the failure of the individual to adjust himself to life, thus he says: [1] " Without exception lack of adaptation is the characteristic of all these patients, and it is this, as well as psychic exhaustion, that causes most disorders." Again: "There are circumstances of life, always the same, which for successive generations set the same problems, which demand difficult acts and which are, for numberless persons, the occasion for a breakdown and mental disease. . . . All the stages of the road of life offer hills to climb and, at such hard ascents, the carriage encounters obstacles and the incompetence and weakness of the poor traveller is made evident." Janet puts down this incompetence and weakness to a failure in psychic force. He admits that he does not know what psychic force is. He says: "The study of electric currents would never have been made, if scientists had always refused to consider their effects, or to make note of their variations, before knowing the nature of electric forces. We should have the courage to speak of psychic forces, to note their diminution, their exhaustion or their growth, before knowing their nature or on what organ they depend." On ultimate analysis, this point of view is not really very much removed from the one advanced in this study of neurosis, but on the grounds of trying to find the simplest explanation

P. Janet, *Principles of Psychotherapy*. London 1925.

for the observed facts, we take up the attitude that there is only one source of energy in the body, namely the combustion of food and tissue, which is brought about by the katabolic process which takes place in the course of bodily metabolism. This energy activates the various organs of the body to carry out their functions, and these functions will be performed violently or weakly, according to the degree of resistance offered, and the expenditure of force necessary to overcome this resistance. Hence the apparent quality of the force is determined, in the view here advanced, by the pattern through which the activity flows, and the quantitative variation by the resistance opposed to it, while Janet would postulate a special variety of energy—the psychic energy, differing from other forms of energy as electricity differs from heat, and this psychic energy varies in the quantity available from person to person.

With regard to the existence of a special form of psychic energy it is of course impossible to dogmatize, but, if we refer to the discussion on this subject at the International Congress of Psychology at Oxford in 1923, we find that the gist of the contribution of Dr Adrian, perhaps the greatest physiological authority on the subject, was that, if psychologists liked to talk of psychic energy, there was nothing to stop them doing so, but there is not the slightest evidence that such a thing exists.

If we consider the matter from the point of view of resistances, we can show by physiological experiment in terms of electric current, that resistance is increased proportionately as the activation has to travel over a greater number of synapses. Hence it follows that complicated neural patterns involving extensive cortical areas and a large number of neurones will, when activated, manifest less violent conations than simpler patterns, and this explains the relative violence of release phenomenon. True, that Janet gets over the difficulty by erecting an elaborate hierarchy of activities, according to the amount of work involved in accomplishing any action, and points out that actions at the level of reflection and prevision involve high tension and the expenditure of much potential if not actual energy. This explains why the neurotic who is blessed with only a small available supply of psychic energy cannot attain to these high-level activities, though he may carry out direct impulsive actions with considerable violence. Janet says : " It must be understood that the accomplishment of acts of a high order, belonging to the order of reflection or of work, whether they be carried out completely or incompletely, is still more capable of bringing on exhaustion and depression than the accomplishment of acts of a lower order."

So far as treatment is concerned, Janet considers that the physician should act as the patient's director, teaching him how he can make best use of his available energy, and how he may avoid useless expenditure. This directorship does seem to be the rôle of the physician, if we do not forget that his duty is to help his patient how to overcome his resistances. Although at one time Janet was antagonistic to psychoanalysis, in his later work he gives his assent to it, with certain important reservations, with which we find ourselves in considerable agreement. He says : " It was necessary . . . to bring to light other memories more deeply hidden, but I had in mind only certain special cases, and, although I advised the search for subconscious memories in these cases, I believed it necessary to guard against discovering such memories, where they did not exist." But, as he says in another place : " I believe it important to eliminate the causes for exhaustion (or as we should prefer to say the manifestations of resistance) that the subject's situation may furnish in his habitual surroundings, and among these, social influences are the most important. It is when one finds no explanation in the actual life of the patient, that it is justifiable to seek into his past life." "Many patients are exhausted, not by the memory of some former adventure, but by the difficulties of a daily life, that is too complicated for their psychic power, and that presents at every turn too many obstacles." "The efficacy of a therapy depends on the diagnosis ; quinine or salvarsan would have the same random effects, if they were applied as psychotherapies are applied. Each psychotherapist praises his own method, which he claims is original, and inclines to apply it to everything, because it cures everything. One moralizes, the other hypnotizes everybody ; one man rests and fattens, another psychoanalyses at random. What would be thought of a physician, who would boast of giving digitalis to all his patients, while his fellow-physician's speciality was the giving of arsenic ? " He therefore thinks that suggestion and persuasion have their place in the physician's armamentarium, but that what really has to be done, is to study the patient and find out where help is needed, and how it can best be given, and with this one cannot but agree, for the psychotherapist ought, so far as is possible, to make himself master of all the methods of mental treatment, and be ready to apply any form which is called for by the special problems of his patient.

G

CHAPTER V

PSYCHOLOGICAL TYPES IN NEUROSIS

It is the duty of the physician, when presented with a case of neurosis, to discover what sort of a personality his patient was before the breakdown occurred, what change the failure of adaptation has brought about, and to what extent he can be restored, if not to his original form, at least to an adequate adjustment to life. In this investigation the physician is helped, if he has some sort of scheme, whereby he can pigeon-hole the various types of personality with whom he meets in the course of his work, provided always, that he uses such a scheme as a means to an end and not an end in itself. There are many such schemes, the most useful in my opinion being that which has been worked out by Jung. Freud's classification, while undoubtedly delineating recognizable types of personality attributes these to the persistence of anal eroticism, urethral eroticism, oral eroticism, and the like. We have already suggested that the Freudians lay too much stress on these eroticisms, and therefore it does not seem advisable to try to work on these premises.

In considering the classification of Jung,[1] we must distinguish between his earlier and later work. Originally he chose two types, the introvert and the extravert, which corresponded as he then described them, to the introverted thinking type and the extraverted feeling type of his new classification. The more elaborate scheme of his later work is a distinct

[1] C. Jung, *Psychological Types* (Int. Lib. of Psychol.). London and New York 1923.

advance and removes several difficulties. In the first place, it relieves us from the necessity of postulating two definite types of introvert and extravert. He now defines introversion and extraversion as attitudes. The four types he relates to the four mental functions of thinking, feeling, intuition and sensation. Whichever of these functions is predominant in an individual determines his type, and this type will be introverted or extraverted, according to his prevalent attitude towards his environment, which may vary from time to time ; so that, although we may say that a person is an introvert, he may be extraverted towards certain objects, and at certain times. Thus a man may be introverted towards his religion, but extraverted towards his garden, while another may be extraverted in health, but become introverted during illness. There can be no doubt whatever that in neurosis, the tendency is for the patient to become more introverted, and this is what might be expected when we consider that a conflict is taking place within the self-regarding sentiment. In this process much cortical activity is involved and therefore attention tends to be directed towards the conflict and not towards the outside world.

The extravert attitude is that, in which the individual is particularly responsive to stimuli of all sorts which come from outside the ego. Therefore the objective aspect of the universe will be that to which attention is mainly directed. Facts, rather than theories, are important and attractive, and action, rather than reflection, will be the direction which is taken by the conative impulses of the individual. On the whole the extravert is a good mixer, he readily attaches himself to others, though he may not make any really close friends.

The introvert attitude, on the other hand, is that in which the individual is particularly responsive to stimuli of all sorts, which come from within the ego. Therefore the subjective aspect of the universe will be of special interest to the introvert

and theories rather than facts attract him. He is a poor
mixer and finds social intercourse rather a trial. He is compensated for this, however, by making really close friends of
those with whom he does find contact. As has been said, the
neurotic of whatever type tends to become more introverted,
the extravert manifesting certain introvert characteristics,
while the introvert becomes more turned in on himself than
ever. On the whole, though this cannot be taken as a universal
rule, hysteria or dissociation syndromes tend to be the form
of neurosis developed by those of extravert tendencies, while
introverts will develop anxiety symptoms or obsessions.

Let us now turn to the various types described by Jung,
though certain modifications of his original description seem
desirable. Jung [1] describes four types—Thinking, Feeling,
Intuitive and Sensational—all of which differ according as the
dominant attitude of the individual is extravert or introvert.
The thinking and feeling types, the rational types, as Van
der Hoop [2] describes them, seem to be organized at a higher
level than the empirical types, the intuitive and sensational.
The principal difference between the rational and empirical
types is that the latter are content to accept the facts of life,
or the impulses they feel within themselves, as they come.
They have no desire to discriminate these, or integrate them
into systems, or control them, so that they come within the
scope of rational laws, as do the former ; and it is just these
functions which are characteristic of full cortical development,
and therefore are higher in the scale. For this reason I would
not regard the functions of thinking and feeling, in the empirical
types, as recessive, in the sense that sensation and intuition
are recessive in the rational types. In the rational type,
sensation and intuition have been superseded for general
purposes but by no means suppressed, so that in certain

[1] C. Jung, *Psychological Types.*
[2] Van der Hoop, *Character and the Unconscious* (Int. Lib. of Psychol.).
London and New York 1923.

situations intuition or sensation is the function that is called upon ; indeed it is only through the rational functions that sensation and intuition can really come to full fruition. On the other hand, in the empirical types, the functions of thinking and feeling have not yet come to full development, and so are only made use of tentatively and occasionally. Since in neurosis, the level of cortical activity is definitely lowered, as a result of the conflicts, which are taking place, it follows that those who are normally of the thinking and feeling types will readily fall down to the empirical level, and lose their capacity for rational reactions.

This classification of Jung's has been criticized as smacking too much of the discredited faculty psychology, but if we try to follow it out from a physiological standpoint this need not be so.

By the function of sensation we mean that the normal sensations acquire a sufficient degree of relatedness to achieve consciousness, and form perceptions, but are not further integrated into abstract concepts, or complicated emotional relationships. Under the term sensation we must include all sensations, whether the result of stimuli coming from the environment or from within the body. I retain the term sensation type because it has been used by Jung, and a multiplication of terms, referring to the same thing, is undesirable ; but it seems to be a little unfortunate to use a word, which has a perfectly definite meaning on one level, to express something indubitably dependent on what is expressed by the original term, but which has acquired a new relatedness, and has emerged at a higher level. It is not pure sensation which this type experiences, but an organization of sensations, so that they emerge as perceptions. These perceptions might be described in our daily press, by the favourite adjective, " sensational," for people of this type are apt to live at a high tension, passing from one " sensation " in the journalistic sense to another. The spontaneous contribution of their inherent impulses, irrespective of response to psychic traumata, is recessive, and only makes itself felt under exceptional circumstances. That is to say, they require something coming from the outside to which they can respond, before action is initiated. When their inherent impulses do initiate action, by breaking away from the usual channels of responses, such action is undiscriminated and uncontrolled, as it has not achieved that degree of relatedness which corresponds to full cortical or conscious control. These people do behave, in response to accidents in the course of their experience, in the way that Freud would have us believe to be practically universal, and their sex impulse, for instance, is either poorly controlled, or repressed by some stronger stimulus from the environment.

If the sensation type is extraverted, he is specially sensitive to, and interested in stimuli from without. Such individuals often achieve considerable powers of discrimination in respect of these, and many artists are of this type, excelling in virtue of this sensory discrimination. As a rule, people of this type are of the class met with in scores at English country houses, interested chiefly in sensuous pleasures in the broadest sense, which include the pleasures of muscular exercise and simple visual, auditory and gustatory stimuli, but they are restrained by tradition, which divides conduct into things which " are done," and things which are " not done." This results in a very definite ethical code, arranged according to the dictates of this tradition, which does not always correspond to the decalogue. Moreover, conduct is frequently dominated by that eleventh commandment, " Thou shalt not be found out." The thinking of these people is superficial, and the only realities for them are facts, and what they call " common sense." Abstractions and metaphysics are quite meaningless to them and simply a waste of time. Their feeling also tends to be superficial, they have hosts of acquaintances, but do not readily make close friends. They say they are deeply moved by events, but alter their lives very little as the result of these " moving experiences," for their own emotions are not firmly established, nor are they well organized, so that they are incapable of real and lasting sympathy. Their chief recessive characteristic is the behaviour dictated by their own " wishes," which is characteristic of the intuitive type. Of this they are desperately afraid, because it usually cuts across the tradition by which they are guided, and leads to a state of confusion from which they see no outlet, owing to the poverty of their capacity for thought. Being a recessive character, the type of reaction is poorly discriminated and controlled, and tends too much to an " all-or-none " behaviour. Hence they are liable at times to violent swings from one extreme to the other, between strictly conventional behaviour and that dictated by their primitive unconscious impulses—behaviour characterized either by a rowdy exuberance of emotional expression, or by crude indulgences in an attempt to satisfy the demands of appetite.

If the sensation type is introverted, he will be interested chiefly in the impressions he receives from within himself, and will react, even to outside stimuli, from this point of view, so that the resultant perception is dominated, chiefly by the influence of the individual's store of images, rather than by pure sense impressions. Much modern art is the product of this type. The sole object in the execution of the work of art is to express how the artist sees a thing. The resultant picture may be, and generally is very different from the photographic impression which the extravert of the same type would experience. Indeed, it may be, that any other person fails to detect any resemblance to the original, but this does not in any way disturb the artist, for how other people see, or feel, or think, concerns him not at all. In their ordinary behaviour individuals of this type being concerned with their own inner sensations, tend to be reserved and withdrawn from life ;

they are irresponsive and apathetic. If they have poor self-assertion, they recognize that they are different from others, since they cannot go out to meet life and enjoy it. Further, they are not well organized and integrated, and therefore they are not sufficient unto themselves. For these reasons, they are apt to develop a sense of inferiority, and fall into a neurosis in consequence. If self-assertion is strong, they may break out into fits of rebellion and aggressiveness, which may take a serious asocial direction. Of such stuff the sufferers from dementia præcox are made. In these cases the world of phantasy is of the highest importance. Here, all inner sensations have free play to work themselves out and gain full satisfaction, so that this false world becomes more important than the world of reality. Even at the best, however, people of the introverted sensation type have great difficulty in expressing themselves, and are usually solitary and morose, too often unhappy in their lives, envying the fortunate lot of the easy-going, sensational extravert.

The person of the sensation type, who develops neurosis, tends towards greater introversion, and consequently the traits of the introverted sensationalist are met with to a greater or less extent. At the same time the patient definitely loses grip of himself and loses confidence in his ability to meet the demands of life, since his trouble is usually due to some conflict with his relation to his community. In view of the fact that his life has been moulded largely in accordance with external tradition and not by any inherent integration of his own, he is very much at sea and very much frightened. He needs a deal of help and direction from his physician, and cannot be left to his own devices at all, since his inner impulses are inco-ordinated and not under control. The physician must try to develop control of these by the force of his own personality, and gradually re-educate the patient, so far as possible, towards rational reactions, and at the same time try to restore him to an environment, where he can find a guidance for his conduct and a satisfactory outlet for his activities, in response to quite definite stimuli of a reasonably simple and beneficial type. Work, congenial if possible, is essential for this type, and it is amongst this class that occupational therapy may succeed without the assistance of any other method.

The second type, termed by Jung "intuitive," is in some sense the antithesis of the sensation type. The latter is susceptible to impressions, and depends on that part of the complex pattern determining behaviour, which arrives, so to speak, from outside the nervous system, by way of the receptors; the former, on the other hand, depends on that part of the complex, which is within the nervous system in the form of disposition. In other words, intuition is the spontaneous expression of the individual's dispositions or "instincts," using the word in McDougall's sense. As in the sensation type, the discrimination and integrative functions of thought and feeling are poorly developed. They do not control the spontaneous outpouring of the impulses, and this type tends to react in the "all-or-none" way, glorying in freedom from restraining logical thought. Nor are their feelings in better way, for feeling, organized into sentiments, is also inimical to intuitive expression.

The intuitive is always trying to find an outlet for his impulses, and the extravert of this type seizes upon objects in the outside world as means to this end. He often perceives association between events which, to others, seem to have little or no connexion, and the future sometimes proves him surprisingly right, but this same faculty may also lead to disaster. The reason for this is, that he approaches these events or objects from a different standpoint from that of any other type. For him, the objects have no value in themselves, but are only important in so far as they can serve the purpose of the development of his own inner impulsion.

This gives a quite different associative link from that employed by the sensation type, and so a different outlook results. Once he has used the object, he tends to drop it entirely, since it has no intrinsic value, though at the time he may have regarded it with the greatest enthusiasm. This applies to persons as well as things, and so he appears changeable and fickle. As a rule, he is not a very dependable person, and prefers to wait until the event arrives rather than bind himself by any plans made beforehand. If the inner impulse, which is seeking expression, is in harmony with the needs of the community, he will, in virtue of his new and single approach, see ways out of difficulties which fill the admiring multitude with awe and rapture. But if this impulse runs contrary to the community's needs, then he will appear to throw over his friends or his nation, and almost deliberately lead them astray. Moreover, impulses of value and impulses with no value may succeed one another with bewildering rapidity, and in truth these civic virtues and vices are only incidental, for all that is of importance to this individual is the practical satisfaction of his own inner requirements.

If the intuitive is introverted, he will not be concerned with practical results. He is more interested in how that which comes from within himself, the product of his own engrams, works, and what it leads to, irrespective of outside objects and events. Most of his activity will be in phantasy, and he will be credited with what is called inspiration. The artist, the poet, the prophet, and the mystic are of this class, and, as was the case in the extraverted intuitive, their value depends on whether their inner impulse is in harmony with other needs. If so, then their poetry and their prophecy is hailed as heaven-sent, but if not, then their effusions are regarded as the vague vapourings of an impractical dreamer. As a matter of fact, inasmuch as the engraphic patterns, on which the mental activity of the type depends, are the product of long ancestral experience, much of value may be forthcoming, and original points of view may be produced, since their archaic nature is little influenced by consideration of contemporary events. So vivid are the inspirations which arise, that the individual does not always recognize them as products of his own mind. This gives rise not only to hallucinations proper, but to impressions that someone else has told him what to say. This is exemplified by many of the prophets of old, who believed that the voice of God whispered His message in their ear.

If this type develops a neurosis, it is usually on account of some definite disharmony of his own impulses, quite irrespective of external events, and consequently it is improbable that any significant psychic trauma, explaining the neurosis, will be found, as is so often the case with the sensational type, and it is rather a waste of time searching for it by elaborate analysis. The patient becomes absorbed in phantasy and is specially liable to wallow in the slough of self-pity, weaving phantasies of what would have happened " if only " things had been different. He sometimes is a difficult patient to treat, because he rushes off on some track, which he is quite certain is the right one ; this may take the form of some quack remedy or a method of cure which he has " discovered." However, the difficulty is, that he does not stick to anything long enough for it to do any good, and so goes round and round, without getting any further. The physician must try to get him to face facts as they are, and not as he would like them to be to suit his own inner impulses, and he must restrain his phantasies. This is very necessary, for so long as these phantasies are out of reach of his actual capacity he never makes any real progress, always wasting time on thoughts of what he would like to do, and never getting anything done. Suitable occupation is useful in this case, but just any work is no use at all, so that unassisted occupational therapy is seldom of much avail. The physician must try to find out where the patient's own natural impulses, founded on his disposition, would lead him, and put him in the way to find contact with life once more along these lines.

The remaining types described by Jung, which involve the functions of feeling and thinking, represent the attainment of a higher level than those just referred to and, as has been pointed out above, their behaviour corresponds to functions associated with the highest cortical development. Two of these functions are discrimination and integration, and Jung's function of thinking is concerned with discrimination, and that of feeling with integration, at a level at which a considerable measure of synthesis of the lower forms of mental reaction has already been achieved. In either type, the lower levels of sensation or intuition may be recognized as dominant or recessive. In other words, the subject may react chiefly to external impressions, or to inner impulses ; but as a rule, these are synthesized into a more or less organized whole. In this way activity depends, not on isolated activations of disparate parts of the total personality, but there is a greater tendency for the whole individual to find expression as a unity. When such synthesis has been achieved, the function of thinking is concerned with discriminating the best method of action, while that of feeling is concerned with organizing the sentiments towards carrying out the required activity. Both of these functions will certainly operate in any individual's mind, for organized activity is impossible without the operation of both the functions of thought and feeling. Yet we say that some people are more addicted to discrimination and thought, and others to integration and feeling leading to action.

Persons of the feeling type are those who organize their reactions with external stimuli, or with their inner impulses, as the case may be, so that their personality is dominated by strong emotions, or, if the feeling involved is more prolonged, by moods. These emotions tend to lead to definite actions, carried out to their logical conclusions. A man of this type will feel the need of a great variety of these emotional patterns which enable him to react to the various situations of his life, and he will put great value on these. So much are these feeling reactions important to him, that he will only value those things which are consonant with his feelings, and will reject everything else, but, if his adaptation is good, his feelings will show such great variety and plasticity that there will be few situations, which he is not prepared to meet. This is specially so, when his attitude is extraverted, for in virtue of this he will be at special pains to adapt himself to outside things and events. He will hedge himself round with organized reactions, which can be called out to meet every conceivable event, and will get on all right until he comes up against the inconceivable event. Then he is at a loss, for having no organization wherewith to meet it, his power of discrimination is recessive and inadequate, and so it is difficult to think out a line of action quickly, to meet the emergency. He will also have a considerable degree of control and understanding, both of his own feelings and those of others. He is never at a loss to recognize what sort of feeling he is experiencing, and will readily estimate the degree of feeling appropriate to the occasion. He will be able to get into close sympathy with others, and his power of suggestion will be considerable. However, he will necessarily prefer pleasurable feelings to unpleasurable, and may be led from this to try to find things as he wants them to be, and thereby neglect the stern truth and be satisfied with the semblance of things in the form of wish fulfilments. This makes him somewhat unreliable as a scientific observer, for he is apt to twist his facts to fit *a priori* hypotheses.

As the extravert feeling type wishes to get into harmony with the outside world, so the introvert wishes to get into harmony with himself. He is inwardly sure of himself, but not well adapted to the outside world, and is therefore critical towards it and apt to be criticized by it. This leads to being misunderstood, and to a difficulty of expressing his feeling to others in ordinary social intercourse. Nevertheless, the harmonious integration of his impulses and perceptions may find expression through poetry and art, in the most delicate way, and this type is often deeply religious, having achieved an inner harmony of emotional reactions, organized round a central belief, which becomes all the stronger because the individual is not concerned with, or influenced by the opinions of the outer world, like the extravert of the same type. The best of this type is the real strong, silent man, who knows what he wants and achieves complete organization of his whole personality towards that end.

Neither the extraverted nor introverted feeling type easily develops neurosis ; indeed the introverted person of this type is peculiarly well integrated within himself, so is naturally not liable to develop conflicts. The extravert of this type, however, may break down if he meets with the " inconceivable event," and in that case will regress towards the sensational type or intuitive type as the case may be. Even so, however, the neurosis is not a severe one, since he has an inherent capacity for integration, which stands him in good stead, and moreover the " inconceivable event " does not as a rule last for long, and so the circumstances which were responsible for the neurosis pass away. These people, if they do suffer from neurosis, often get well without treatment, " by their own effort," as they think, giving themselves somewhat undeserved credit, since, what has really happened is that their difficulties have automatically passed away. Hence they are apt to be somewhat intolerant of their less fortunate brethren, who cannot rise by their own unaided effort, and whose difficulties persist.

As has been said above, the function of thinking is concerned with that of discrimination, knowledge is its province, and classification its business. However, facts are not the only materials which serve as the subject of this discrimination ; impulses and sensations also come within its purview. The man of the thinking type is concerned with differences, with right and wrong, with this and that, and so has ethics, metaphysics, and much of philosophy for his special field.

The extravert of this type is concerned in his scheme of classification with the objects of outside experience, which he calls facts. Further, he will tend to classify them according to the accepted standards of the community. He will tend to collect an enormous quantity of facts, and cram them into the pigeon-holes already provided for him. When these facts do not fit into these pigeon-holes, he is apt to become extremely dogmatic about them, asserting, with no little heat, that they do fit, because they ought to fit ! This is so when the type is evolved from a basis of the function of sensation. The chief activity will be directed towards amassing experiences, and these people are good scientific observers, though they may require the corrective of an introvert attitude in properly arranging the facts. If the basis is the function of intuition, the extravert thinker will be interested in the classification of the feelings and impulses of other people, and he will find his interest in history and criticism. He may also achieve eminence in co-ordinating the work of others, as a business organizer. If the extravert thinker is possessed of a narrow outlook, his tendency to force facts into certain accepted categories makes him bitterly hostile to everything which comes outside the limits of these categories, and so he becomes intolerant and bigoted. He is dry and dull as his feelings are recessive, and, as he cannot pass the bounds of the class in which he places himself, he tends to be a conservative of the die-hard type. The recessive feelings may at times find expression, and if so, they will be uncontrolled and ill-adapted, giving rise to violent outbreaks of temper or other emotional reaction. This is especially liable to be called out in these people if someone does not agree with them, and their rigidity tends to make them carry their theories beyond their legitimate boundaries, so that they insist on a universal applicability ; as for example, the ultra-Freudian, who derives every activity from infantile sexuality because he has become impressed with the importance of this latter in certain relationships.

The introvert thinking type moulds the scheme of classification according to lines worked out by himself. If such an individual is of high-grade mentality, this is valuable, because the scheme of classification he adopts will be elastic and adaptable. If evolved from a basis of sensation, he will test his observed facts against his scheme, and his scheme against the facts, so that they become adapted to each other. If, however, his mental capacity is less adapted, the scheme of classification he works out may be of little value, and may lead him into the most egregious errors.

If he deals with intuitions, he classifies and criticizes his inner impulses, and in so doing may destroy his usefulness, for he is always considering how and why he does things, and never gets them done. This type of thinker is eminently introspective, and is more interested in the abstract than in the concrete. He more readily understands and sympathizes with other people's faults and difficulties, for he does not classify them according to accepted principles, but recognizes them as subject to the variations of impulses that he knows so well in himself. For themselves, these individuals are reserved and shy, and do not readily express their opinions. If they do so, they will appear to the extravert, as caring too little for those of others. The opinions of others, indeed, are objective phenomena, for which men of the introvert type do not care, but the feelings of others are of much greater subjective interest, and so come more within their purview. Their shyness and reserve make them awkward in company, and the lack of control of their recessive feelings makes their emotional reactions inconsistent and unpredictable. The rules which their subjective function of thought lays down for them lead, however, to the formation of ideals which they often fail to live up to. This induces a feeling of inferiority for which they try to compensate by phantasy formation. If this is applied to the ideal of their own character and behaviour, an ever-widening gulf may be formed between reality and phantasy, with disastrous mental conflicts and subsequent neuroses. In any case, this is the type of man who plans before he acts, and who may fail altogether if his plans miscarry, so that in future he never gets beyond the planning stage, lest he should subject himself again to the indignity of failure. However, if his plans succeed, he will often carry out his actions with remarkable persistence and success.

The discriminative function of the thinker is responsible for a liability to neurosis, in spite of the high level of his personality. A peculiarity of neurotic symptoms is the facility, with which part of one pattern is split off and reattached to another. This is discussed at greater length in Chapter VII, and it will be seen there, that it is the discriminative function, which is chiefly concerned in the process. The thinking type, when he has developed neurosis, is always much troubled by the uncontrolled and excessive manifestations of his feelings, and one of the chief duties of the physician must be to help him to a realization of their true significance. It is often found that he has previously prided himself that he never showed his feelings under any circumstances, but investigation shows that this was not due to real control but rather to repression, the affective activity being held in check and cancelled out by opposing patterns. With the development of neurosis he can no longer achieve this repression, since conflicts are

H

present on a larger scale and fatigue diminishes the available cortical activity at his disposal. To his disgust, therefore, he finds that he weeps at nothing and reacts violently to everything. The physician must explain all his symptoms to him, for the thinker demands explanations and is much comforted thereby. He is sometimes helped by well-chosen psychological literature and, if put on the right lines, can often do a very great deal by himself in the way of unravelling his symptoms, owing to his power of discrimination. Sometimes the patient is liable to rather unaccountable regressions, generally due to emotional upsets which throw him right off his balance, depriving him, for the time being, even of his power of clear thinking.

These brief sketches are no more than indications, and every physician will have to work out for himself the scheme of personality types which he finds most useful, but I believe that the working out of some such scheme is of real use in elucidating the problems of the neurotic.

CHAPTER VI

THE ANXIETY STATES

THE form of neurosis described in this chapter is very common, and the name anxiety state may be applied to those cases in which the symptom of anxiety or angoisse is the most prominent and significant feature of the illness. A vast deal has been written about this symptom (angoisse or Angst), which is present at some time or other in all neurotic illness. Its manifestations, which are both mental and physical, are the invariable accompaniment of conflict within the personality. The absence of this symptom in certain hysterical cases is referred to and explained in the discussion on hysteria on page 172 but, as will be seen there, the exception is more apparent than real. Pathological anxiety is an intensification of normal anxiety—itself a conflict within the personality between the emotions of hope and fear with concomitant physical manifestations. The most characteristic of these is a spasm or irregular muscular action of the diaphragm, some-times referred to by patients as " their insides turning over," " a sinking in the pit of the stomach," and so on. At the same time palpitation and other cardiac irregularities, sometimes accompanied by anginous pain, are very common, while pains in the head, giddiness, and swishing noises are often complained of. Less universally present symptoms are nausea and even vomiting, peristaltic irregularities, diarrhœa and tenesmus, " spasms " of all sorts, vaso-constrictions with cold extremities, asthma, air hunger or suffocation and disturbances of sweating salivation and other secretions, which may rarely be unilateral. The mental symptoms comprise intense apprehension and fear, sometimes with no specific object, but often with the emotion attached rather loosely and expressing itself as a dread of death, heart disease, insanity, etc. These more definite anxieties are however secondary, and the results of suggestions emanating from one or more of the physical accompaniments. Sleep is practically always disturbed and nightmares are present.

It is unnecessary to enumerate further the symptoms of " angoisse," since they have been described so often, especially by the French. It is much more important to try to explain under what circumstances this syndrome of symptoms is experienced by the patient and the physiological processes on which it depends.

We may first consider the Freudian conception of anxiety. The original Freudian teaching with respect to the symptom (Angst) was, that in all cases it resulted from unsatisfied sexual desire,[1] more especially from sudden enforced abstinence or from the practice of *coitus interruptus.* The view, which I wish to put forward here, is that it is the necessary concomitant of any conflict between emotional dispositions within the personality. In our investigations of neurotic patients, we are forced to the conclusion that many of them, if not most of them, do suffer from conflicts in respect of their sexual life. That this conflict does frequently concern itself with the problem of masturbation and marital relations is undoubted. In the first category the conflict between the impulse to masturbation and the biological and ethical influences, which restrict it, is often intense and the practice may be given up, as a result of fear of imaginary consequences, rather than because the patient understands the situation and has achieved real control. Under such circumstances there may be marked consequent anxiety. The Freudians say that this anxiety

---

[1] Breuer and Freud, *Studien über Hysteria*, Vienna, 1916.

is due to the giving up of this form of sexual gratification and, if they are absolutely honest, as some of them are, in this respect, they must recommend resumption of the practice or indulgence in some other form of sexual gratification in order to cure the symptom. Experience shows, however, that unless all ethical inhibitions are removed at the same time, the anxiety is enormously increased by any attempt on the part of the patient to follow such advice. If such ethical inhibitions are removed, the anxiety disappears, not because of the physical gratification, but because the conflict is resolved. Admittedly, such conflicts are difficult to resolve, unless some more satisfactory outlet of the sexual impulse is possible, for sublimation is all very well in theory, but the establishment of complete control over crude physical appetite cannot always be achieved at once. In the second category, where conflict is concerned with emotional reactions towards marital relations, it is again the resolution of the conflict and not the gratification of physical desire, which removes the anxiety, and here advice and council about such matters is often of great help to the patient.

Again, it is often found that there is no sexual component in the conflict, yet marked anxiety is experienced. The familiar conflict during the war, between duty and fear, was attended by the most definite anxiety, and this distressing symptom was removed, when the conflict was solved, quite irrespectively of any sexual connotation. For the theorist to insist that such anxiety was due to deprivation of sexual satisfaction, as a result of war conditions, was proved over and over again by actual facts to be a piece of self-deception whose only object was to fit facts into a special mould.

Again, in civil life, the attempt to show that the anxiety of the widow, when bereft of a husband, was due to deprivation of sexual gratification may be shown to be wrong in many cases. For example, a widow of 52 was left with three sons at school and a somewhat complicated estate to administer, with a fellow-trustee aged 23 and with no older relatives whatever to advise or help her. She suffered marked anxiety, and various ill-defined phobias for trivialities, because she failed to adjust herself for the time being to the new circumstances of life. She was the subject of a definite conflict between her self-depreciation, which had been fostered under the indulgent and dominating personality of her husband, and her sense of duty and maternal responsibilities in respect of her boys, and as this was resolved she lost her anxiety. On the other hand there had been no sexual relationship for many years before her husband's death, so there was no deprivation and there had been no anxiety up to the time of his death, for this symptom had only developed when the new conflict had arisen. The argument, that in every case of anxiety sexual deprivation of some sort has been discovered, is not convincing, for it is probable that under modern civilized conditions very few people, if any, do not suffer or have not suffered from some sort of sexual deprivation. Economic stringency is responsible for late marriages and restriction of families, and the principles of birth control are not yet sufficiently widely known, or satisfactory in practice, to allow preventive measures to be practised, without some want of satisfaction or mental conflict. Therefore, some of those suffering from anxiety may be so suffering from mental conflicts arising in their sexual life, which actually do depend on sexual deprivation, but it is suggested that the anxiety is due to the conflict and not to the deprivation. For the rest, it will be found that they are suffering from conflict, but, if they are questioned, it will not be difficult to obtain a story of some sort of sexual deprivation ; however, the same will be found to be the case with normal people, who are not suffering from conflict or anxiety.

When we turn to the physiological aspect of anxiety, we

notice that all the symptoms complained of are due to activity of the vegetative nervous system and that this activity is diffuse, ill organized and often contradictory in its apparent purpose. For example, the patient will complain of sweating at the same time as tightness in the chest. Sweating is due to a stimulus of the secretory nerves to the sweat glands, which is a sympathetic function and part of a pattern of vegetative activities, which are directed towards enabling the animal to undergo hard muscular exercise. The special function of sweating in this pattern is partly to enable heat to be dispersed by evaporation from the surface of the body, thereby preventing the body temperature rising, as it would as a result of muscular activity, and partly to assist in the excretion of the toxic products of this activity. In the same pattern of vegetative activity, we find that the sympathetic function in respect of the lungs is to dilate the bronchi, thereby encouraging free aeration, more rapid oxygenation of, and withdrawal of carbon-dioxide from the blood and at the same time reducing body heat. In the anxiety state, however, we find constriction of the bronchioles, a vagal activity completely antithetic to sympathetic action. Other examples of this disintegrated contradictory action of vegetative function could be mentioned, but the above will serve as an example.

It is suggested that anxiety is the direct result of two or more emotional patterns in conflict. When an emotional pattern is prevented from expressing itself in the normal form of motor activity, proper to the motor section of the pattern, it is a matter of common observation, that the vegetative part of the pattern is activated more violently and less coherently. For example, if we are frightened and can run away, we take to flight with our motor functions and vegetative functions acting harmoniously, our legs running, our skins sweating moderately, our hearts accelerated and our bronchioles dilated, but, if we are prevented from running away, these vegetative activities become excessive, we sweat abnormally and our heart goes off in " palpitations " and so on. In the situation postulated of conflict of emotional patterns, since their normal activities would be contradictory, they counteract each other's motor activity and, as a consequence, the vegetative activity is increased in violence. But, just as the motor activities are in opposition to each other, so are these vegetative activities, and so we have a disintegrated contradictory pattern of vegetative tensions, which are experienced as the physical manifestations of anxiety. These vegetative activities, however, have not only a physical aspect but also a mental aspect and this, corresponding to the complicated patterns of visceral tensions, comprises a complex subjective pattern of unpleasure, which the French term angoisse and the Germans Angst, and to which we have given the name of anxiety, though it probably does not exactly correspond to the emotion anxiety (anxieté). This concept is admittedly sketchy, so far as the details of the experience of anxiety are concerned, but we must remember we are very far from understanding the exact relationship of sympathetic and vagal activities and their mental correlates. None the less, it does seem to cover the occurrence of this peculiar experience in the circumstances of mental conflict, whereas other explanations do not seem to be founded on physiological principles or on adequate evidence.

Among the most characteristic symptoms of the anxiety states are insomnia and sleep disturbed by nightmares. The researches of Pawlow and the conclusions drawn by Adie in his study of narcolepsy seem to point to certain discoveries with regard to sleep.[1] Firstly, sleep would seem to be a process identical with inhibition, the latter is " a partial and strictly localized sleep, confined within narrow limits by an opposing process of stimulation, while sleep is inhibition which has

[1] W. Adie, *Idiopathic Narcolepsy* (*Brain*, XLIX. 1926), p. 257.

spread throughout the cerebral hemispheres and to subcortical centres." Sleep will be encouraged by reducing stimuli, and thus quieting points of excitation in the cortex, and conversely, it will be prevented by the occurrence of fresh stimuli and the " building of a new point of excitation in the cortex." There is a good deal of evidence that lesions in the region of the optic thalamus—midbrain and pituitary-tween brain systems—influence sleep by diminishing, increasing or altering its rhythm, as happens in *encephalitis lethargica*. This region is also known to be associated with vegetative function and emotional reaction. With these considerations in mind, it is not difficult to see how mental conflict interferes with sleep and that insomnia is a common symptom in the anxiety states. Further, if a fresh stimulus is likely to interrupt sleep, it is not difficult to see how dreams may arise and cause disturbance. It must be remembered, that when two emotional patterns are in conflict, they counteract each other but do not inhibit each other, just as when both flexors and extensors of the wrist are activated simultaneously, no movement occurs, though neither group is inhibited in the physiological sense. If inhibition were to occur under such circumstances, the wrist would eventually become flaccid, but in the process, one or other side might temporarily gain ascendancy and the wrist flex or extend accordingly. Similarly, when inhibition becomes sufficiently general for sleep to ensue, the counter-action of the one pattern relaxes and the other is enabled to enjoy partial expression. Such expression, however, cannot be in any way direct, for this would " build up a fresh point of excitation in the cortex and the individual would awake." As Freud has pointed out, I think correctly, this is avoided by an indirect or symbolic expression, which is achieved by the activation of an associated pattern. A dream of greater or less complexity then occurs, and this is associated with greater or less emotional intensity in accordance with the degree of side-tracking which has taken place, the emotional intensity being in inverse proportion to the complexity of the ideational content. It is noticeable however, that with waking, the counteraction of the opposing pattern is often rigidly reinforced and repression is reimposed, so that the dream content is promptly forgotten. This process is analogous to the action of an electro-magnet. Directly contact is made, the magnetic attraction ceases and contact is broken ; directly contact is broken, magnetic attraction is again present, and contact is made, and so on indefinitely. Similarly, directly inhibition (sleep) allows pattern A to escape from the counteracting influence of B, and A finds some sort of expression (a dream), a new excitation starts and inhibition tends to be disturbed, and counteraction is reimposed by B.

So many volumes have been written on the subject of dreams, that it is not proposed to discuss them at length or to give any examples. It may be well, however, to recapitulate the process of dream formation. It has been shown that the old ideas of dreams being due to indigestion or other physical stimuli are not adequate, either to explain their occurrence or to indicate treatment, for, however thoroughly the physical well-being of the patient is cared for, the dreams still continue. Furthermore, the physical theory does not explain why, on one occasion, the dream may relate to one series of events and, on another occasion, to quite a different matter. It is not disputed that such physical stimuli may and do act as instigators of the dream, but it is contended that the psychological mechanism of the dream is the important part, and a thorough understanding of this will enable the physician to help the patient to get rid of his nightmares.

The study of dreams in general reveals the fact that they always express the fulfilment of some conative tendency— a tendency towards the completion of an impulse, a striving towards, or away from, an object or situation, or, expressed in more general terms, the fulfilment of a wish or fear. Thus in a dream the patient may find fulfilment of something which he has been wishing for or something which he has been dreading. Such a wish or fear may be either conscious or unconscious ; that is to say, the subject may be perfectly aware that he does wish for or dread the object in question, or he may not realize it at all or only partially realize it, but nevertheless his whole mental activity is being influenced by it. Experience shows us, that the less complex the mentality of any individual is, the more directly will dreams express his wishes or fears, and the more conscious these wishes and fears will be, so that we find that the dreams of children, primitive and simple-minded people, are much easier to analyse and explain than those of people whose brains are very highly developed.

In analysing and explaining dreams, certain rules should be attended to. In the first place the dream must never be taken as a whole, but each part or section must be considered as complete in itself and studied separately. It must be remembered, that in the dream the material which underlies it is condensed to a very large extent ; consequently the various incidents may represent very much more than is apparent to begin with. Secondly, the phenomenon of displacement must be kept in mind. By this is meant that the people or incidents, which are represented in the dream, may not be the actual people or incidents to whom the dream refers. Similarly, incidents, which seem extremely important in the dream, as narrated by the subject, may have very little significance indeed, while others, which are slurred over, are found to be the really important elements. Thirdly, the setting of a dream tends to be intensely dramatic and bears the same sort of relation to the events which it represents, as a Drury Lane melodrama does to the lives of ordinary people. Lastly, there is a tendency for subsequent accounts of dreams given by the patient to differ widely from that given immediately on waking, although he has not the slightest desire to deceive. This I proved in the case of my own dreams, by writing them down immediately on waking and again several hours later. On comparing the accounts, I often found surprising discrepancies, although I had conscientiously tried to put down only what I remembered. In investigating any dream, it is therefore very important, that it should be narrated by the patient as soon as possible after he has dreamt it, and however he may subsequently correct himself as to his impressions of the dream, the first account should be taken as the one which most closely represents the dream as it was dreamt.

The extent to which the analysis of dreams is useful in the treatment of a neurotic patient is a matter of some dispute. If he is suffering from a persistent nightmare, there is no doubt that it is very well worth while to find out its meaning and significance in relation to the difficulty experienced by the patient in his adjustment to life. By so doing, not only will the nightmare be exorcised, but considerable light will be thrown on the conflicts of the patient. As a rule, such nightmares are not very difficult to elucidate and no great time is expended in the process. It is otherwise, however, in the case of casual dreams, and it seems to me that the very long and elaborate analyses of dreams, sometimes carried out by the orthodox psychoanalysts, do not always produce results commensurate with the labour and time expended. It is often useful, however, to get the patient to collect and narrate his dream material, as it often happens that sooner or later he does have a dream, which throws a flood of light on his conflicts and difficulties, without any elaborate analysis being necessary. It is important, however, that the patient should not take the collection of dreams too seriously, for, if he suffers from the scrupulosity which characterizes some neurotics, he may lie awake all night in a state of dread, lest he forget some part of a dream.

Partly as the result of the insomnia, and partly as the result of the fact that much of the energy available for mental activity is taken up in the continued activation of opposing patterns, the neurotic patient complains of fatigue and exhibits the signs of inefficient cortical activity. He is easily tired by mental and physical exertion of any sort and complains of having none of his old energy or enthusiasm for life. At the same time he suffers from headache, which usually takes the form of a dull ache, varied from time to time by neuralgic pains. If the night has been disturbed by nightmares the patient will wake with a headache, but, as he gets more controlled as the day goes on, the headache is relieved, only to come on worse as the patient gets tired again towards evening.

Cortical inefficiency is seen in the inability to concentrate his attention, to marshal his ideas and to remember things when he wants to. These failures depend on the inefficiency of the highest functions of the cortex—integration, discrimination and reference in time and space. Patterns cannot be integrated into constructive wholes, differences cannot be discriminated and images and perceptions cannot be referred accurately to their proper time and space relationship. The anxiety case frequently states that he has lost his memory, but this is not so, for his power of recording impressions is not lost and the reactivation of pattern which constitutes recall does take place, but not at the time at which the patient requires the recall. Then no effort on his part can recall the lost memory, but later it all comes up quite clearly, perhaps while he is in bed at night.

Depression is almost universal in these cases. It would appear, that this results from the absolute failure on the part of the patient to understand the nature of his illness. This condition is often accentuated by his realization that many of his physicians do not understand it either.[1] He feels ill and experiences many symptoms both physical and mental, and yet he cannot put his hand on what is the matter. He tries to tell his doctor what is wrong, but only succeeds in being loquacious, without being definite or convincing. He is given many forms of treatment which do no good. Too often he has been moved from one place to another, from central hospital or nursing home to convalescent home, and vice versa. He has alternated between unappreciative abuse and sloppy sentimentalism. He becomes convinced that he has a disease which no one can understand, and from which he will never recover. He sees his chances in life slipping from him. Financial and family cares overwhelm him and he sinks into a slough of despondency, from which it is difficult to arouse him.

To such a man, the appreciation and understanding, the robust and helpful sympathy of efficient psychotherapy comes as a ray of sunlight through the fog of his despair, and it is as well to add at this point, that treatment cannot be regarded as complete, until the patient has been placed in a suitable occupation, so that he can face the world with renewed courage and cast off the trammels of his former despondency.

General irritability is another symptom of the loss of control, and it is a very common complaint among neurotics that they have a period of great distress during the early morning, which is apt to be worse after a good night than after a bad one. Janet [2] drew attention to this phenomenon and attempted an explanation on the basis of psychological tensions, a concept which is hard to reconcile with the standpoint taken up here. Obviously, to the patient this symptom is a distressing paradox, for the physician is continu-

---

[1] Cf. Millais Culpin, *One Hysteric and Many Physicians* (*Brit. Journ. of Psych. Med. Sect.*, III.), 1923.

[2] P. Janet, *La Tension Psychologique* (*Brit. Journ. of Psych. Med. Sect.*, 1921).

ally telling him that sleep is all-important, and the better he sleeps the worse he feels in the morning. If we study the morning distress complained of, we generally find that the patient wakens rather early, feels uncontrollably restless and irritable both with himself and others. For instance, a man with a somewhat severe neurosis in the early stages of his recovery, when he was beginning to sleep better, would wake up any time between four and six a.m. and feel extremely irritable and restless. He would wake his wife and abuse her for not taking him away, and make all sorts of wild statements about himself and her. He would then walk over the town, once or twice went down to his physician's house, rang the bell, purposing to tell him he could not go on any longer, but went away again before anyone could answer and, after considerable agitation and distress, went home for breakfast. Shortly after he had eaten this he began to feel calmer and better. Clearly, we have to deal with diminution in control of ideational, emotional and motor activity. It is a commonplace that in sleep the control of all our functions is lessened and, if sleep is not too deep, ideational, emotional and even motor activities manifest themselves in considerable confusion in the form of dreams. It is not meant to imply that dreams are without method or meaning, but only that the activity of dreams is not so controlled or integrated as the activity of waking life. Under normal circumstances, provided the waking is natural, that is to say, that we have had our sleep out and wake up of our own accord, presumably when the natural rhythm comes full turn and our refreshed activities overcome the inhibitions placed on the flow of afferent impulses to the cortex, the restoration of full cortical control is immediate. However, if we are forcibly wakened out of sleep, before our tissues have recovered from fatigue, we are apt to exhibit considerable irritability and absence of full integration and control. The neurotic is a person whose cortical control and integration is for the time being poor in quality, easily exhausted and readily upset, and it would seem that instead of the immediate restoration of full control this is only slowly achieved. Furthermore, this failure to re-establish control may be due to an actually feeble and ill-nourished condition of the cortical cells, for the effect of breakfast consisting, as it usually does of such cerebral stimulants as tea and coffee and assimilable carbohydrates, is often remarkable. Further, as the day proceeds, fresh stimuli induce more and more points of activity in the cortex, and so, as Pawlow has shown, sleep and inhibition are abolished and more complete control is possible. If the patient has spent a wakeful night, the abolition of cortical control is never so definite and complete as is the case during sleep, so that in the morning there is relatively little or no re-establishment necessary, and consequently there is no such feeling of extreme restlessness and distress, though, as the day wears on, the patient is not so well as he is on those occasions on which he has had a relatively good night followed by the morning irritability. This symptom is sometimes the cause of very considerable distress to the patient, but he should certainly be encouraged, for it is only a phase in the process of recovery. As his general control and adjustment improves, the period during which he is unable to establish control becomes shorter and shorter, until he regains the prompt response of the cortex in re-establishing its functions, once he wakes from his full night's rest.

A similar failure of full cortical control accounts for a very common symptom in anxiety states, namely the feeling of unreality. Janet drew particular attention to this symptom and described it as a loss of the function of the real. This function he described as that which made the difference in our feeling for reality as opposed to phantasies and simulacra, in our feeling for the present as opposed to the feeling for the

future or the past. This might be felt in respect of external
things, or in respect of the ego itself, " quand ils disent qu'ils
ont perdu leur moi, qu'ils sont à moitié vivants, qu'ils sont
morts, qu'ils ne vivent plus que matériellement, que leur
âme est separée de leur corps, qu'ils sont étranges, drôles,
transportés dans un autre monde." [1] Many neurotics complain
of this, either permanently or intermittently, and it often
causes them very considerable distress indeed, chiefly because
they do not understand it and consequently think it may be
a symptom of insanity. As usual, Janet's description of this
symptom could not be bettered, but simply to say that it is
a disturbance of the function of the real does not get us much
further, for there is no attempt to define the processes on which
this function depends. It would seem that the explanation
is to be found in the dissociation and disorganization of control,
and the failure of discrimination consequent on the defect of
highest cortical function. I think some analogy may be drawn,
if it is not insisted on too far, with diplopia. Here the subject
perceives two images of, say, a candle flame, and may not be
able to distinguish the real from the false, *i.e.*, the one corresponding in space with the real candle flame and that of the
displaced image, so the neurotic cannot discriminate clearly
between phantasy and reality owing to the failure of integration of cortical function, just as diplopia is due to failure
of integration of binocular vision. There is more than this,
however, for the sense of reality in an object depends on the
degree of attention paid to it, and the neurotic is notoriously
poor in his powers of attention. Active attention depends on
the organization of patterns into systems with an affective
appeal. These patterns are in relation to one or more of our
dominant sentiments. For instance, we can as a rule fix
our attention without any effort on our ambitions, our loves
and hates, and it is in virtue of the organization of the pattern

---

[1] P. Janet, *Les Névroses*, p. 353.   Paris 1919.

I

in relation to these sentiments that the so-called fixation of the attention is possible. In the anxiety patient, however, the ordinary dominant sentiments, particularly that of self-regard, do not secure the control of the rest of the personality, as they do in the normal, since the influence of the conflicting and counteracting patterns prevents this. Consequently the objects of ordinary life have no affectively organized pattern, to which to be attached. For this reason they remain as perception patterns, which are activated, but, not being organized with affective disposition, lack the "function of reality" which Janet describes. With the resolution of the conflict, this disability is removed, and so the sense of reality is again enjoyed by the patient.

Certain fears are very commonly experienced by the anxiety patient, and require mention : these are the fear of insanity and the fear of committing suicide. This brings us to the point, Does the neurotic commit suicide ? A most important question for every physician. If we accept as a definition of the neurotic, that he is a person who has failed to adjust himself towards life, *but is still trying to do so*, the answer is No. So long as life is a reality which is striven towards, the barrier of the self-preservation instincts, to say nothing of moral and religious scruples, is too strong to be overcome by the impulse to shirk life or to damage the ego. The question which then arises is, Does the neurotic who has failed to adapt himself ever abandon the struggle ? It is difficult to be dogmatic on this point, but my own experience is that however inadequate and unsuccessful the efforts of the patient to face life, the true neurotic, *i.e.*, the personality which emerges from the " bundle " of patterns which we have sketched above, scarcely ever does abandon the struggle and certainly never does, if he has the least confidence in anyone as able and willing to help him in his struggles. That is to say, if any positive transference is established between the patient and his physician, or whoever is his mentor, the risk of suicide may be completely discounted. Since one of the best ways of establishing this transference is to assure the patient, who is the victim of obsessive thoughts that he might commit suicide, that there is no chance of such a thing happening, I have no hesitation in saying that the physician should encourage the patient to discuss the matter fully and should never express a doubt on the subject at all to the patient. Nor is this in any way humbugging or deceiving him, for, if the patient will only trust and believe in the physician, there is no risk whatever of his doing harm to himself. The next question that arises is, Does the patient ever lose interest in life altogether, so that his patterns are no longer set towards adaptation to life, but in some other direction altogether? In other words, Does he become insane? My belief is that he does not, that insanity involves quite a different emergent personality and that one does not pass into the other. But there can be no doubt, that in the early stages of dementia præcox, manic depressive insanity, paraphrenias, paranoias, and even in general paralysis of the insane, the correct diagnosis may be a matter of great difficulty, and many persons are labelled neurotic, who are really insane. This I believe accounts for the frequent newspaper reports of neurasthenics, who have committed suicide, which strike such terror into our neurotic patients, lest they go and do likewise. While this difficulty in diagnosis is a decided stumbling-block to us physicians, and while we have probably all made mistakes, it does not alter the principle, and should only serve as a stimulus to us to learn more about the early symptoms of insanity. If a neurotic patient is feeling particularly under the weather and feels that his disability is not attracting the attention and sympathy it merits, he may commit acts, which he tries to persuade himself amount to attempts at suicide, but which deceive no one else. For example, the patient quoted on page 170 with hysterical paralysis tried to make out that she had attempted to kill herself by throwing herself over a parapet, but as there was a drop of less than three feet on the other side, it was not very convincing. Contrast this with the historic, if somewhat legendary sailor, who tried to kill himself on three separate occasions, by jumping over the Dean Bridge in Edinburgh. Again a neurotic was very depressed one morning while shaving and slightly cut the skin of his throat with his razor, whereupon he rushed from the room and roused the whole institution by shouting that he had killed himself. Contrast this with the true case of a very feeble old woman, with scarcely strength to wield a razor, who accomplished her purpose at the seventy-second slash. The latter was undoubtedly insane, the former was neurotic, and while one would hesitate to hand him a razor and ask him if he would not like to finish the job, I believe that such a callous rejoinder to his exhibition would be attended by no danger to the patient.

If actual suicide does not occur in a neurosis, the idea of suicide, appearing occasionally or obsessively in the consciousness of the neurotic, is extremely common, and I believe this to be a symptom of doubt and hesitation and in no way to represent an impulse towards the act. The fear of the lay public and of many members of the medical profession of the harmful effect of the idea of suicide entering the patient's mind is based on the erroneous ideomotor psychology, which was so prevalent at the end of the last century. Superficially, it seems not only likely, but obvious, that an idea coming into our minds impels us to carry out an action which is appropriate to it, but the more recent dynamic psychology of McDougall and Freud has shown pretty conclusively, that action depends on the set of the great inherent dispositions, and that an idea *per se* has no power to set our muscles in action. We do not fly because of the idea of danger, but because activation of

afferent channels, which mentally lead up to the perception
of a dangerous object, acts as a stimulus to the neural pattern
or engram laid down as our inherent disposition, our instinct
of flight.   Indeed, the idea of danger in the abstract conspicuously does not cause us to fly, nor does the idea of suicide
cause us to cut our throats.   Therefore, I believe that there is
no reason at all, why we should not discuss these ideas of
suicide fully and frankly with our patients ; indeed, unless
we do, we are not likely to help them to divest themselves of
such ideas.   We have laid it down, that neurosis depends
on an inability to adjust towards life, whether the difficulty
lies in adjustment to our own special reactions, or to the circumstances of our environment.   Here then we have a conflict presented to our neurotic : " Shall I make this great effort
of adjustment and endeavour to adapt the ego to the demands
presented to it, or shall I give up the struggle altogether ? "
The apotheosis of the first is the ultimate success and defeat
of all difficulties, which is constantly present to the neurotic,
but unfortunately only in phantasy, because it cannot be
achieved owing to the impediments imposed on him by the
lack of harmony within his personality.   Similarly, the apotheosis of the second is death, *i.e.* suicide, but this is also in
phantasy, because of the impediments imposed by conflict,
but in this case also, because the inherent impulses to self-
preservation and adaptation to life cannot, in the neurotic,
be overcome.   We have already pointed out that the normal
and the neurotic are set towards adaptation to life, and therefore self-preservation has enormous value and suicide is not
carried out, whereas in the insane the set is away from adaptation to life.   " Life " and reality cease to be of importance for
the latter, and therefore self-preservation loses its value and
suicide is more easily accomplished.   It may be said that in the
normal individual suicide does not appear even in phantasy,
while in the neurotic it is common.   This is to a large extent

true, but can any but the most blatantly self-satisfied extravert truthfully say that no occasion has ever arisen in his life when things seemed too difficult, and the idea that a quiet slipping out of existence would be the easiest solution of the problem has never entered his mind ? To the neurotic, in his state of conflict and poor integration, ideas representative of parts of his personality comprising individual impulses, which are not co-ordinated into a harmonious whole, are a commonplace, and so it is not surprising that the idea of suicide is frequently in consciousness.

Still another aspect of this question presents itself for study, for the idea of suicide is not always the passive phantasy of escape from struggle, but may be rather an active antagonism against the self. That the sufferers from the anxiety type of neurosis, at any rate, are centred upon themselves, is a self-evident fact. Freud has expressed this as a regression to narcissism, a state normal in infancy, when the self is the object of love. Care must be exercised, however, not to press this theory of regression too far. Certainly the infant is entirely concerned with the gratification of his own desires and impulses, and to a considerable extent finds means of gratifying these simple desires in his own person, but the infant does not enjoy the full power of reflective thought, whereby the ego is clearly differentiated from the universe. For the infant the universe is merely a vague continuation of himself, but the neurotic does not lose this reflective differentiation, at any rate under the conditions to which we are referring. To put the matter in another way, the infant has not formulated a self-regarding sentiment, in which the ego is the nucleus of emotional dispositions having reference to it, since he has not yet differentiated the ego to form a sentiment. On the other hand the neurotic emphatically retains the self-regarding sentiment, although this is in a state of conflict instead of being organized harmoniously together, as is the case in the normal. In the neurotic the emotional dispositions are alternatingly ambivalent with regard to the ego. At one moment, the ego is the object of love and approbation, at another of hate and despite. The apotheosis of the latter emotional set would of course be destruction of the ego, and this is possible in phantasy but not in reality, since the disintegration of the personality is not sufficient to overcome the set towards self-preservation and adaptation to life. Obviously this hate and impulse to destroy the ego lends force to the suicide phantasy, which would lack vigour, if only expressing a withdrawal from the struggle. This accounts for the more violent suicide phantasies which are sometimes met with. It is to be noticed, however, that there is an ambivalence of emotion within the self-regarding sentiment. That is to say, there is a concomitance of opposite emotions and not a mutual exclusion, so that the stronger the self-hate the more violent the reactionary self-love. When this gains ascendancy, the patient experiences a horror and dread of suicide, and it is in this form that the suicide phantasy sometimes becomes fixed as a definite pattern of an obsessive fear lest he commit suicide.

The conflict between desire for life and fear of death is well exemplified by those neurotics, who are continually telling the physician how they propose to end it all, and almost in the same breath beg him to examine their heart, as they are so afraid that it might be the seat of disease and that they might drop dead at any moment. These incompatible ideas are kept in " logic-tight compartments," so that they do not seem in the least incongruous to the patient, but they are of course simply further examples of expressions of conflicting patterns, which lack that integration which would cancel them out in the normal individual.

The same explanation accounts for the frequency with which the neurotic talks about getting well, but is unwilling or unable to make that last effort to do so, which is so necessary.

Very slight acquaintance with neurotics, however, will convince the physician that the patient gains very considerable advantage from his illness in avoiding tasks and duties in life, which are difficult and irksome, and, if the acquaintance with the problems of neurosis is very slight, the physician may assume that the patient is perfectly aware of this and is exploiting his illness for his own ends. When he gains more experience, however, he realizes that this exploitation of illness is not so conscious and deliberate as at first sight appears, but that the whole business is bound up with the conflicting emotional patterns, and that it is not so much the simple duties, which will have to be faced, that are dreaded, as the situation, which was the origin of the neurosis from which he has been suffering.

The fear of insanity, which often accompanies the fear of suicide, depends to a large extent on the suggestions of others and on auto-suggestions from the patient's preconceptions as to the meaning of symptoms. Many people think that if an illness is said to be mental, this necessarily means that the person suffering from it must be insane. This is of course nonsense, just as it would be nonsense to say that if a person had something wrong with his chest, he necessarily suffered from tubercular disease of the lungs. Still more people think that if a patient suffers from certain symptoms, which are known to be prevalent amongst the insane, that person must be insane. Most neurotics suffer from depression and some may have hallucinations, but this no more necessarily means insanity than a pain in the stomach means cancer. However, the neurotic patient is so mystified by his condition, and gets so little help, that he becomes frightened and wonders if perhaps, after all, he may be going out of his mind. He is afraid to mention such a fear, and still less under these circumstances will he talk about his ideas of suicide, lest people should confirm this horrible suspicion and shut him up in an asylum.

In treatment it often takes a certain time before the physician has gained the confidence of the patient sufficiently to enable the latter to confess to this fear of insanity, but the reassurance on this point does take an enormous load off his mind.

With regard to the treatment of the anxiety states, if the fundamental factor in the production of the symptoms is mental conflict, this must be dealt with, if cure is to result, and any other treatment which may be given, must be in the form of symptomatic remedies and recognized as such. Such symptomatic remedies, however, are not to be despised altogether, and it often happens that the judicious administration of the milder hypnotics, such as the various urea derivatives, helps to give the patient sleep and, diminishing the fatigue and restlessness, enables him to co-operate in the main part of the treatment, better than he could otherwise do. Similarly, sedatives are sometimes of service and, in my experience hyoscine is useful in allaying the most severe exacerbations of angoisse.

As to the resolution of the conflict, this will require some sort of mental analysis, and the exact method used by any physician will probably depend on his own personality, and the contribution of training to that personality. So much has been written on the methods of psychoanalysis and its various derivatives, that there is no lack of guidance for those who can take advantage of the written instructions of others. It will be found, however, that as in most other things, it is personal experience which gives skill and sureness in technique. All I would say in conclusion is, that, in my opinion at least, while much of the material which has to be obtained from the patient is unconscious, the patient is aware of more than might be suspected, if the Freudian theory of complete repression and the absolute unconsciousness of the origins of neurosis were whole-heartedly accepted.

CHAPTER VII

OBSESSIONS

In addition to the general symptoms of anxiety described above, certain major symptoms are met with in some patients, which may all be grouped together under the term obsessions. To understand what is meant by this, it is necessary to have a clear definition. The following, which we owe to Bernard Hart, seems adequate :

" An obsession is an idea, action, or fear, intruding itself into consciousness in a manner which is felt by the patient to be irresistible. It does not fill the field of consciousness or dominate it indisputably. It is an incomplete and imperfect thing, recognized by the patient as being in itself inadequate and unsubstantial."

Investigations show that obsessions depend on some complex, which is not integrated with the rest of the personality, and so is more or less dissociated, and is also more or less repressed. This complex, or the intellectual, emotional or action pattern belonging to it, is presented in consciousness in an irresistible manner, without any rational introduction, and, in so far as this pattern is itself well-defined and definitely integrated, the urgency with which the obsession enters the field of consciousness is considerable. At the level of consciousness, however, it finds no firm associations ; it cannot become integrated within the personality and influence the total conduct ; the mental processes are not correlated and are not sufficiently comprehensive, and hence the obsession does not fill the field of consciousness or dominate the mind indisputably as do the somnambulistic and allied states which will be discussed in Chapter X. Thus, as expressed in the last part of the definition, it becomes an incomplete and imperfect thing, recognized by the patient as being in itself inadequate and unsubstantial.

In the light of this definition, to what extent can we admit certain phenomena commonly described as obsessions to be true obsessions ? There are three false uses of the term, and these should be clearly differentiated. The first is memory preservation. For example, it is said that a mother is obsessed with the memory of the death of her child. This does not fulfil our definition, for, while it may not dominate the mind, it is something which is very real to the mother. These persistent memories should rather be termed preoccupations.

Secondly, there are dominating tendencies and ideas, which may be normal or pathological. For example, a man is said to be obsessed by his ambition to succeed in the world. This ambition may or may not completely dominate the mind of the individual, but it is certainly something which he regards as perfectly real and substantial. These dominating ideas may be pathological, as in those which are met with in paranoiacs, who are said to be obsessed with the idea of escape from their persecutors. They are not only real to the patient, but they truly dominate his mind. Associated with dominating ideas are dominating fears, which are met with often enough in neurotics, as well as in normal people. These differ from phobias, which are true obsessions, in being real to the patient, since they are founded on perfectly adequate causes and may be removed by pointing out to the patient that his fear is groundless. Such a dominating fear is the fear of insanity, which may be caused by hallucinations often met with in neurosis. A hallucination is a neurotic symptom, but the fear of it is not, and once the patient is made to understand why he has hallucinations, and once he is shown that he is not becoming insane, this fear disappears. Another example of the same thing is seen in the case of a man who is said to be obsessed with the fear of drowning when he goes to sea in a small boat. Here again the fear is real ; it has a perfectly adequate cause and is removed directly the voyage is over. Somewhat different, but still not a true obsession, is the dominating fear of the paranoiac of his persecutors, for this fear clearly dominates consciousness and influences every action.

The third group is that of impulsive actions. These are met with in normal people and in the insane, but quite rarely in neurotics, but they again are not true obsessions. The impulsive action is met with in those people who are commonly called impulsive ; they suddenly perform an action, without there being any apparent rational antecedent for it. Part of an instinctive pattern comes into consciousness, and if not opposed by any contrary instinctive pattern, action takes place before doubt can arise, which will inevitably occur, if the subject attempts to think out the advisability of his behaviour. In the insane this process manifests itself in the sudden suicidal and homicidal outbreaks, which occur from time to time. Such actions dominate the consciousness, and are essentially real.

Janet [1] has pointed out, that obsessions are often connected with subjects and objects which are held in particular horror by the patient. Thus a man at the age of 16 had visited a so-called museum of anatomy, where various models and specimens of the effects of venereal disease upon the human body had been laid out, with a maximum of crudity. They made such an impression on his mind that he had gone about thereafter, in particular horror of these diseases. Later in life, he developed a severe neurosis, in the course of which he had

[1] P. Janet, *Les Obsessions et Psychasthenie.* Paris 1889.

auditory hallucinations, or rather pseudo-hallucinations, for he knew that the voices were not real. In these hallucinations he seemed to hear a conversation about himself, in which the following sentence was reiterated over and over again : " Oh, yes, he is quite a smart lad, but he has the pox."

In obsessions, ideas of what the patient holds most sacred are often mixed up with others which he holds in abhorrence ; thus Hart describes the case of a young girl, who cannot think of God without immediately associating this idea in her mind with some sexual or excretory idea. In such a case, we have a clear example of the underlying basis of deficient correlation, for, in the structure of the normal mind, the idea of God would be integrated with the religious pattern and the idea of excretion with a physiological pattern. In the obsessional case these ideas have, so to speak, broken adrift and become attached to the wrong pattern, because of some early association between them, which became imbued with intense emotional tone and was repressed. Obsessions are often connected with sacrilege, especially amongst those who are brought up in a strict religious environment, and with certain crimes, such as suicide, homicide and theft. Much controversy has raged round the question, whether such a patient will carry out a crime about which he has an obsession. The general consensus of opinion is that he will not do anything that really matters, but Raymond has pointed out that exceptions occur in the case of kleptomania and dipsomania. Suicide has been discussed in Chapter VI, and the same argument applies to the more serious crimes. The case of kleptomania, however, is somewhat different, for investigation shows that the impulse to steal depends on all sorts of conditioning of the instinct of acquisition with sex, revenge and other patterns. The acquisitive instinct is fairly strong in all of us, and it is probable that in the predisposition of the individual, who becomes a kleptomaniac, it is particularly influential.

The force of herd tradition, even when this is intensified by the superaddition of other emotional patterns against taking the possessions of others, is not nearly so strong as the opposition to the taking of life. Hence, in this conflict, if acquisition is conditioned and intensified by other patterns, we may expect to see the balance tipped quite frequently on the side of crime. Similarly in dipsomania, we have still further attenuated herd tradition pitted against the desire for excitement and new emotion for which the neurotic always longs. Moreover, the neurotic seeks the abolition of self-criticism, which alcohol insures, and so the impulse to drink often gains the day. Furthermore, the true dipsomaniac attack represents a definite effort to cloak or resist some intensely unpleasant complex, which is overcoming resistance and so becoming conscious. Common obsessions, illustrating the process of conflict, are the patient's shame of himself and shame of his body. These depend on the sense of inferiority and the strengthening of the self-abasement pattern, which is very characteristic of the neurotic. In the course of his phantasy he builds himself castles in the air about himself or his personal appearance and then realizes with a sense of despair, that they are not for him, and so starts the conflict between the patterns of self-assertion and self-abasement that constitutes the dominant factor in the mental processes of so many neurotics.

From these conflicts develop the hypochondriacal obsessions as to health. Such obsessions are frequently sexual and grafted on them will often appear hysterical symptoms, which have been suggested by the patient's ideas of his own ailments, such as impotence, pains and aches of all sorts.

Associated with such definite obsessions are obsessive questionings, which are derived from the patient's general loss of the sense of reality. They may begin by abstract metaphysical enquiries and then become true obsessions characterized by the recurrence of the most absurd and futile questions, such as, Why are the trees green ? Why is the sky blue ? and so on.

It is obviously impossible to describe all separate varieties of obsession, but it is necessary to give a short description of the true obsessions. The first group is that of obsessive ideas, which may be systematized or diffuse. Amongst the systematized ideas are the abnormal associations, such as those already quoted in the case of the young religious girl who always associated God with something unclean. More important are the hallucinations of the neurotic. These should really be termed pseudo-hallucinations, as the patient is usually quite aware that the things he sees or hears are not real. The false images, which the patient projects into space, are found to be connected with the conflicts which are causing his condition, much as are his dreams. For example, a soldier who suffered from a pre-existing neurosis, markedly exaggerated during the war by the conflict between his ideas of duty and his intense distaste for army life, had the following hallucinations : On going along a road by himself he saw, on more than one occasion, two men in hospital blue walking in front of him. They left the road, as if to hide and wait for him, but when he reached the spot, they had disappeared. The hallucination was sufficiently vivid for him to be able to recognize the men as two patients, who had been with him in another hospital sixty miles away, and his insight was sufficient to enable him to realize that they could not have been there. As a matter of fact these two men had taken him from this hospital to the neighbouring town, where he had been told he would be court-martialled for disobeying orders. He had keenly felt the irregularity and indignity of this, especially as he realized that any disobedience on his part was due to his illness, which was in no way understood. The hallucinations thus depended on the painful memory of this experience, and his dread of going back to suffer similar indignities at the hospital he had recently left. All that was necessary to banish these hallucinations was to show the patient their true significance. Hallucinations may be extremely important, since they are liable to instil in the patient's mind a real fear of insanity. He realizes he is seeing things or hearing things, which do not exist, and so jumps to the conclusion that he must be going mad, and the treatment of neurotics sometimes does nothing to dispel the idea.

In addition to the systematized obsessive ideas we have diffuse obsessive ideas, which are termed ruminations. These are characterized by want of action rather than action, and exemplify particularly well the neurotic's inability to make up his mind to one course of behaviour. At times the neurotic will set out to do some simple action—to buy a present perhaps; then he is assailed by doubts. Should he buy this object, which is cheap but is not so good, or that, which is rather more than he had meant to give ? All degrees of such a reaction exist, from what would be regarded as a perfectly normal hesitation to the fruitless expenditure of several hours. This rumination is often closely connected with the mania of perfection, as when the patient stands before a letter-box and ponders whether to post his letter or not ; he is sure there is something he ought to have added to it, and yet he ought to post it, or his friends will get anxious for news of him. Again, in extreme cases he sits wondering whether he should tie his shoe-lace in a knot or a bow for most of the morning.

Amongst the systematized obsessive actions must be mentioned manias and pacts. These manias are impulses to carry out some particular action in a perfect and satisfactory manner, but being obsessions the actions never are perfect and satisfactory, and so tend to be repeated again and again. A few examples of manias will illustrate what is meant. It should be noted that these manias have nothing to do with the mania of manic-depressive insanity, and it is a pity that the two conditions should have the same name.

A very common mania met with in these obsessive cases is the mania of perfection which may be exhibited in all degrees of elaboration. In the most severe cases the patient will spend hours performing some simple task such as rolling up his umbrella or cleaning his nails, because he cannot satisfy himself that it is sufficiently well done. Such symptoms are dependent on the conflict between opposing patterns, which prevents the action being carried out to a satisfactory conclusion and the transference of attention to something else.

In these cases the patient feels impelled to carry out the action, while fully aware of its futility and absurdity, and the actual performance or otherwise of such actions will depend on the propelling and resisting forces of the patterns on either side. The senseless manias, such as continually washing the hands, or going to look if the gas is turned off, depend essentially on a displacement of feeling tone from some pattern which is intimate and painfully important to the patient, to one which is of no importance. It is a partially successful attempt to avoid conscious contact with the painful pattern, and the mechanism of the production of such manias is essentially the same as that described below as responsible for the production of phobias.

Pacts form another group of systematized obsessive acts. Most individuals have indulged in pacts at some period of their lives, which is not surprising if we recollect that neurosis is but an exaggeration of a normal reaction. By a pact is meant the performance or avoidance of some action, accompanied by a vague feeling of impending disaster, if the action is not duly performed or avoided. Familiar ones are the avoidance of the cracks in paving-stones when walking along the street, or the feeling that one is impelled to touch every lamp-post. We may remember Christopher Robin and the Bears and the

K

Squares. Such are referred to by the old writers as *délire de toucher*. A notable example from literature is that of Jean-Jacques Rousseau, who felt that overwhelming disaster would overtake him if he did not hit a tree with a stone, and he spent hours in carrying out this action ; it is interesting to read, however, that he never ran any risks of missing, for he always chose a large tree and took aim from very close at hand. Such pacts are very common amongst neurotics. The symptom fits into our conception of obsessions very well, for the patient is aware of the foolishness of his actions, yet always shirks the task of bringing himself to book and asking himself the value of his performance. He can never sufficiently collect his thoughts to find out what it is he expects will happen if he does not do the deed, nor why he should do this particular thing and no other. The real reason is that like manias the pacts bear some symbolic relationship to a painful complex.

Tics are often included as systematized obsessive actions among the symptoms of obsessions, but it would seem that they are more properly described as hysterical, though they occur very frequently in association with other obsessions.

The diffuse form of obsessive action is the emotional crisis familiar to every one as an attack of 'hysterics.' The ebullition of emotional expression, accompanied by diffuse and purposeless motor activities is too familiar to need description, and this symptom, at any rate, is the very essence of inco-ordinated mental activity. It frequently serves as the origin of a true hysterical fit, the seizure becoming more and more epileptiform, as the enquiries of friends and doctors as to the nature of the attack suggest to the patient an elaboration of his symptoms.

The third variety of obsession is the obsessive fear. In this case the systematized and diffuse forms may be considered together. The systematized obsessive fear comprises the various phobias which used to take up so much space in the

older text-books and exercise the authors' ingenuity in invent-
ing new Greek names. Diffuse obsessive fear is the familiar
anxiety or angoisse which we have seen accompanies all
unresolved conflict. This underlies all the obsessive fears
and consists in a nameless, inexplicable dread, which is accompanied by many of the physical expressions of the emotion of
fear : "The dark feeling of mysterious dread which comes over
the mind, which the lamp of reason, though burning bright the
while, is unable to expel." (Borrow). It may be manifested
as a diffuse fear occurring persistently or at intervals without
definite cause, or it may occur only when the patient is forced
to perform a certain action or bring himself into a certain situation. In this latter case the fear is systematized, and the patient
is said to have a phobia for the action or situation which produces the angoisse. Such situations may be of all varieties,
and there seems no point in translating descriptions of them
into Greek and appending the affix phobia, thereby creating a
new disease or at any rate a new symptom, such as the agaro-
phobia, acrophobia, and claustrophobia of the older writers.

It will be evident at once that these symptoms fit extremely
well into our conception of obsessions. As in the case of all
obsessions the patient is perfectly aware that his fear is groundless, yet he cannot so regulate his thoughts as to discover
how and where it arose nor of what it is he is actually afraid.
These fears, moreover, can be shown to depend on repressed
memories and conflicts. For example, a patient who had a
phobia of heights was able to trace it back to a fall off the mast
of a ship at the age of 18. Sometimes a close investigation of
a phobia will show that it is related to a more definite situation
than appeared at first. For example, a man complained of a
phobia of the dark, but investigation showed that it was only
dark tracts of road surrounded by trees which caused him
angoisse, and this was traced back to an occasion many years
previously, when he had been attacked by a native who had

been hiding behind some trees. This close investigation of the exact limits of a phobia is often of the utmost value from the point of view of treatment, and it is always advisable in dealing with obsessions to delimit and define them as accurately as possible. A phobia, however, essentially depends on some repressed mental factor. For example, a patient had a very painful experience, in which he was discovered by his fiancée in a compromising situation, although as a matter of fact he was innocent of any deflection from the path of virtue. In spite of his protestations the engagement was broken off, and as a result he no longer cared for his morals and for a time lived a loose life. A year or two later, however, he formed an attachment for another girl, and, coincident with the time of his discovery that he wanted to marry her, he developed claustrophobia. This fear of closed places was confined to situations where he could be observed by others, such as music-halls, restaurants, and the like. Enquiry elicited the fact that when he realized that he wished to marry the second girl, the events of the past few years came up before him with painful intensity and he worried greatly, as to how they might affect his future prospects. He shirked facing the problem, as he found these thoughts so very painful, but instead tried to forget them ; in other words, he endeavoured to repress the conflict unsolved. It is to be noticed that the most painful memory was that of being found out in a situation from which he could not escape, for this had wrecked his former engagement, and, in order to escape contact with this specific memory, he unconsciously detached the dread, which belonged to this particular event and reattached it to a more general situation, in which he felt himself observed in a place from which he could not escape. Directly this was made clear to him the phobia disappeared.

To generalize from this particular example, a phobia consists in a detachment of the halo of emotional tone properly belonging to a painful, intimate and definite mental process B, and reattaching it to a more general and less intimate situation A. The process comprises a partially successful attempt to avoid contact with the painful mental situation B.

From the physiological point of view the chief interest in obsessions lies in the detachment of one part of a pattern and its reattachment to a different pattern. This is an important feature in the development of many neurotic symptoms. It is specially noticeable in hysteria and will be referred to in the next chapter. An inkling of how this takes place in normal behaviour is given by a study of the experiments on the behaviour of the chimpanzee, carried out by Köhler and quoted by Koffka,[1] who has been kind enough to discuss this matter with me in personal correspondence. One of the " cleverest " of the animals was in his cage, in which was a tree with several branches, while outside the cage was placed a banana a foot or two beyond his reach. After several unsuccessful attempts to reach the banana, he eventually broke a branch from the tree and fished the banana within his reach. It was evident that since this " intelligent " action was only possible for the " cleverest " of the apes, that this represented just about the highest level which could be reached.

The process consisted in the mental detachment of branch from the pattern tree and its reattachment to pattern food. As Koffka has pointed out, these patterns differ in the mind of the ape inasmuch as the tree pattern is emotionally quite indifferent, while the banana pattern was " tense with desire," since the ape was hungry and the banana was a most succulent and desirable means of releasing this tension. All are agreed that instinctive patterns are potent to modify conduct, so that we have a situation which we might roughly describe as one in which there was no particular cohesive tension in

[1] M. Koffka, *The Growth of the Mind* (Int. Lib. of Psychol.). London and New York 1924.

pattern tree, while there was considerable "magnetic" activity in pattern food. Be that as it may, only the highest-grade cortical functioning amongst the apes was able to split up pattern tree from being a whole. This power of splitting up of patterns must depend on the discriminative function of the cortex, which we recognize as a more or less late development. Sir Henry Head [1] has pointed out how the discriminative sensation of posture is represented almost entirely in the cortex, while the almost purely affective sensation of pain is represented in the thalamus. With the development of discriminative function therefore, we have the power of splitting up patterns into their component parts. The branch can be discriminated from the tree by this process but then comes the feat of reintegration. This again is a high-level process and is familiar enough in other cerebral fields. For example, the action of flexing the fingers, at one stage of evolution and of individual development, subserves the grasping reflex and very little else, and all the fingers flex together. Later, however, there is a discrimination of these movements, fingers move separately, acquire new integrations with other finger movements, till in the accomplished pianist, we have the most remarkable digital dexterity, derived from the discrimination and reintegration of primary finger movements. This process in the chimpanzee is therefore a simple example of a mental process, which is probably of great significance in the study of intelligence.

We must now try to compare this with what happens in the obsessions, and I think we shall find that, though the behaviour of the chimpanzee throws light on the obsessions, the latter are regressive processes, while the former is a progressive one.

Let us take examples of obsessions and try to understand how they arise.

Firstly, the girl who had an obsessive association between the idea of or word God and the sexual act, so that whenever

[1] Sir H. Head, *Studies in Neurology.* Oxford 1920.

she thought of or spoke of God obscene words obtruded themselves into consciousness. This depended on two patterns,
which had come into association quite early in childhood,
one representing an attraction towards sex and the other a
repressing religious pattern, involving fear of the wrath of God.
Although these were in opposition, they conditioned each
other in the same way as the instinct of the chick to peck at
any bright object is conditioned by the bitter taste of a red
ladybird, so that in future a bright red object is avoided.
Thus ' sex '—' wrath of God ' were associated for the future,
but this complex in turn came into conflict within the personality, with a shame pattern that such things should have
occurred in her experience, complicated by a self-preservation
pattern, which protects the ego from the unpleasant complex.
These patterns largely cancelled each other out so far as
conative activity was concerned, but the tension involved
intensified the unpleasant affect. The revulsion against sex
had been very strong and for a time had dominated it and held
it in subjection, but later with the intensification of the affective
value and consequent facilitation of the sex pattern, the conflict had become more intense and neurosis had resulted.
The discriminative function of the cortex allowed the patterns
to be broken up into their component parts, but not into their
original component parts, the cleavage being in the opposite dia-
meter. We may represent the process diagrammatically thus :

$$\left(\begin{array}{c} \text{sex} \\ | \\ \text{attraction} \end{array} \right) \qquad \left(\begin{array}{c} \text{God} \\ | \\ \text{wrath} \end{array} \right)$$

Conditioning then takes place, so we have

$$\left(\begin{array}{cc} \text{sex} & \text{God} \\ | & | \\ \text{attraction} & \text{wrath} \end{array} \right)$$

Fresh discrimination takes place during the conflict thus :

$$\text{(sex—God)}$$
$$\text{(attraction \quad wrath)}$$

and while the self-preservation shame pattern succeeds in holding the affective portion in check, the associated sex-God idea manifests itself in consciousness as an obsession, though there is no attraction in the sex idea or cognizance of wrath associated with God. Since the sex—God association is itself obnoxious to the personality, new secondary conflicts and tensions arise, which account for the insecurity and inadequacy of the obsession and the unpleasant affect accompanying it. We can see here therefore that the process is analogous to that which subserves the behaviour of the chimpanzee, but while the latter is progressive and constructive the former is merely a subsidiary effect of a partial cancellation of two patterns in conflict, and the obsession serves no useful purpose, not even that of relieving the difficulties of the patient, because this is done, inadequately it is true, but so far as is possible, by the restraining " censoring " pattern.

Allied to this condition is the obsessive repetition of words and numbers. Patients suffering from anxiety neurosis frequently complain that they find themselves repeating words and numbers which apparently have no meaning or purpose. As to the meaning of these, it may be possible to establish some connexion between such numbers or words and subordinate patterns in the personality, but this is scarcely worth while, since observation shows that they are a cloak to cover up the emergence in consciousness of a pattern which is painful to the patient. Thus for example a neurotic patient had behaved in a way which was not in accordance with his ego ideal, and this gave him a good deal of trouble at the time ; later it sunk into oblivion, but with a further temporary relapse this complex again became troublesome. At first this was not fully conscious, but for some nights the patient complained of repeating words and numbers. Then the old incident came up into full consciousness and the repetition of words ceased. With the persuasion to face the incident and adopt a definite attitude towards it, improvement continued. It was clear that the words were a more or less fortuitous substitute for the repressed complex, which was almost but not quite sufficiently free from restriction to emerge in consciousness. A certain degree of organization with the rest of the personality is necessary for the emergence of any pattern in consciousness, and the repressed pattern, in this case, is not so definitely dissociated, that activation may not spread to it from other patterns of the personality at any moment, unless there is some side-tracking. Rhythmical repetition is a common feature of activity at all levels up to a certain point, from cardiac and respiratory function upwards to the well-recognized repetitive activity of the young child, who, for example, will hum the same tune over and over again to the great discomfiture of his adult neighbours. We see therefore that the tendency for the tail of one phrase in a pattern to be the starting-point of activity for its head is a well-established habit at an earlier phase of existence. We have seen that regression to a lower method of behaviour is characteristic of the neurotic, and this would seem to explain the side-tracking of activation from an unwelcome pattern by means of repetitive activity in respect of relatively indifferent words and numbers.

To remove this symptom, it is necessary to unmask the complex, which is hovering on the brink of consciousness, though of course this may be only one link in a long chain of repressed material on which the neurosis depends.

The next obsession is that of an unmarried woman, who had a cleaning mania, being compelled to wash her hands and clothes over and over again, lest the slightest contamination should cling to them. This originated from an illicit love affair with a married man, which filled her with shame and loathing of herself, and especially of her body, which was kept out of consciousness by her self-preservation " censoring " pattern.   Here then we have sex-attraction pattern and shame pattern in conflict to begin with, then sex dominated by shame, for the patient was now frigid, and shame partly cancelled and held in check by the censoring self-preservation pattern.   The idea of uncleanliness and the incessant action of washing was detached from the original pattern of sex-shame, and appeared in consciousness unattached and inadequate to relieve the tensions engendered by the conflict, although this is the real purpose of the conative activity. Here we see then a rather striking contrast with the chimpanzee behaviour, in which the detached part of the pattern by its reintegration enables the animal to relieve the tensions of hunger successfully.   On the other hand the washing mania is regressive and inadequate, since it is not adjusted to the whole tense pattern, most of which is cancelled out and held in check, but not met and integrated within the personality.

A further example may be quoted of the phobia of the dark referred to above.   In this case investigation showed that the situation which had given rise to the condition was as follows : The patient had been coming along a road by himself, when on military service in India, and when he got to a particularly dark part surrounded by trees, he had been attacked by a native and taken by surprise ; he had lost his nerve, taken to his heels and fled for his life.   Later, he had been filled with remorse and shame at having shown the white feather before the native, and the incident had been repressed and forgotten, though the conflict had been manifested by a phobia of the dark.   Here we have again an example of discriminative splitting of a pattern, but this time the emotional part is manifested in consciousness, while the ideational and conative parts are largely kept in check.

The question as to why the form of obsession—phobia —mania—obsessive idea, should vary from case to case is an interesting one, but one which my experience is too small to enable me to answer, but I strongly suspect that further investigation will show that the differences depend on the variations in personality types discussed in Chapter V. For example, phobias will not tend to occur in the feeling type, who can control and adapt their feelings, while obsessive thoughts and manias will more readily occur in these—the manias in the sensation type and the thoughts in the intuitive type. Again obsessive thoughts will not tend to occur in the thinking type, though phobias may readily do so. This, however, is mere speculation and, since the number of definite obsessive cases coming under observation is necessarily small, it may be some time before this can be determined.

Considerable controversy has raged over the question as to whether cases of obsession should be certified and confined, or not. Cases of recent origin most certainly should not, for under adequate psychotherapeutic treatment, they should be restored to health. In the more severe cases, which have persisted ever since childhood, treatment is apt to be extremely laborious and unfortunately frequently fails in the end. These cases are not a danger to themselves or to the community, but may be a considerable nuisance to their friends. Most authorities, however, are agreed that certification is not justifiable, unless the patient is really incapable of supporting himself, and his relatives cannot or will not look after him. Such patients suffer from many symptoms which are familiar in psychoses, such as hallucinations, illusions and the like. The obsessional case, however, cannot be said to have delusions properly so-called and he has insight into his hallucinatory images. Therefore we cannot categorically describe him as insane, especially as he is certainly still trying to adjust himself to life.

CHAPTER VIII

HYSTERIA

HYSTERIA is a condition in which symptoms are present, which are induced by suggestion, under circumstances in which the patient, either temporarily or permanently, is failing to adapt himself to life. I suggest this somewhat clumsy definition of hysteria, because I believe it does cover the facts. During the war, there was some controversy as to the nature of hysteria. Charcot had been the first to clarify the mysterious manifestations, which had been referred to under this term since the earliest times. He disabused men's minds of the causal efficacy of a " peccant womb," if only because the same symptoms appeared in men as in women, but he concentrated his attention on the more bizarre and dramatic manifestations as exhibited by his show patients. The perfection and constancy of these clinical pictures was perhaps as much due to Professor Charcot as to the original malady of the patient, for, as Hurst has shown,[1] the so-called hysterical stigmata are the direct result of suggestion and can be produced and removed at will. Janet, in his lectures on the Major Symptoms of Hysteria,[2] intensified this attention on the more severe manifestations of dissociation, such as somnambulisms, fugues and multiple personalities.

Freud, meanwhile, had concentrated attention on the psychogenic nature of hysteria, classifying as psychoneuroses,

---

[1] A. F. Hurst, *Seale Hayne Neurological Studies*, p. 21. Oxford 1918.
[2] P. Janet, *The Major Symptoms of Hysteria*. New York 1907.

conversion, hysteria, anxiety hysteria, fixation hysteria and obsessional neuroses, while neurasthenia, anxiety neurosis and hypochondria were classified as actual neuroses. The difference between these two groups was supposed to lie in the fact, that in the psychoneurosis the present symptoms were the direct, or more often indirect expressions of past psychic experiences, while in the latter, the cause was operating coincidently with the symptoms. In any case, the point, on which stress was laid, was that the underlying mental state is the important factor in hysteria. Until this had been dealt with, any attention directed to the actual symptom was held to be a waste of time, and efforts to remove the symptom, even if successful, were merely skating over the surface of the problem, whereby the physician might acquire a bubble reputation, but the patient was not really benefited. Then came the war, with its manifold examples of hysterical symptoms, ranging from paralyses of fingers or toes to blindness and deafness, from facial twitchings to convulsions and even apparent coma. Babinski[1] had previously recognized that such symptoms were the result of suggestion and, for the most part, were curable by counter-suggestion, while Hurst[2] went so far as to state : " Apart from actual hysterical symptoms, there is no underlying physical or mental symptom or group of symptoms, which precede or accompany them or persist after their disappearance, and to which the term hysteria can be applied. . . . The only possible definition of hysteria is this, the condition in which symptoms are present, which have resulted from suggestion." This certainly seems going too far, for we are all exposed to suggestion, but we do not all exhibit hysterical symptoms. None the less, I believe that the nature of the actual hysterical symptom does depend on a suggestion, operative at the time of its onset, but that the

[1] J. Babinski, *Exposé des Trav. Scientifiques*, p. 203. Paris 1913.
[2] A. F. Hurst, *Seale Hayne, Neurological Studies*, p. 109.

increased suggestibility and partial dissociation, which charac-
terize the mental state of the patient at the time when the
symptom is initiated, are due to a failure of adaptation within
the personality.

If we adopt my definition, it is necessary to be quite clear
as to what is meant by suggestibility. McDougall [1] defines
suggestion as " a process of communication resulting in the
acceptance with conviction of the communicated proposition,
in the absence of logically adequate grounds for its acceptance."
Following this, we might define suggestibility as a readiness
to accept propositions with a conviction which is not justified
by logic and reason.

Formerly, suggestibility was regarded as something abnormal, but McDougall and others have very properly shown that
every individual is possessed of this to a greater or less extent.
It is an innate tendency of mankind, and like all other innate
tendencies in man, it is greatly modified during the mental
growth of the individual and in the process of the formation
of his character. Drever [2] has pointed out that suggestibility
is very closely bound up with another innate tendency, that
which McDougall has termed the " instinct " of self-abasement,
if indeed it is not a special manifestation of that disposition.
It is quite obvious that the person with a marked degree of
the opposite tendency, of self-assertion, will not be readily
suggestible, and later we shall see how this operates in the
incidence of hysterical symptoms. We find in every child a
certain degree of suggestibility, which is dependent on the
relative preponderance of the dispositions of self-abasement
and self-assertion, but it is noticeable that compared with
adults, children are markedly suggestible. This suggestibility,
which is a factor of great utility in education, is gradually
modified, till the normal adult reaches his condition of low

---

[1] W. McDougall, *Social Psychology*, p. 97.   London 1917.
[2] J. Drever, *Instinct in Man*.   Cambridge 1917

suggestibility. The young child is extremely dependent on others for his physical requirements, such as protection and nutrition. This demands that self-assertion should be in abeyance and self-abasement in the ascendancy, but as his physical powers grow, the child finds that he can do things himself, and his self-reliance increases. Such self-reliance is a complex sentiment, but its basal factor is self-assertion. As suggestibility consists in readiness to accept propositions with a conviction which is not justified by logic or reason, it follows that the stronger the reasoning powers and the more readily they can be brought to bear on a new situation, the less will be the suggestibility of an individual. But in order to reason about a subject, we must have knowledge about it, and the knowledge must be well organized and well arranged in our minds, if we are to apply it to the new situation. The young child has no knowledge and is therefore unable to resist suggestion, but with increasing knowledge he is more and more able to throw the light of reason on the suggested material. The better arranged and organized is his knowledge, the more rapidly can reason be exercised and the less suggestible will he become. As a result of this organization of knowledge, systems of ideas are built up, perhaps themselves originating from suggestions in the past, but buttressed in the present by all sorts of proofs, which at least satisfy the subject himself. Such systems constitute a man's moral, religious, political and other convictions, which form strong points in his mental field and are specially immune from outside influence. McDougall has pointed out that the least suggestible man is " the wide-awake, self-reliant individual of settled convictions, possessing a large store of systematically organized knowledge, which he habitually brings to bear in criticism of all statements made to him."

In considering the neuroses in general, the dissociation and disorganization of the highest cortical functions as a result of conflict have been pointed out, and, under such conditions, suggestions influence the patient more easily. Hence neurotics are more suggestible than normal persons. When these higher cortical functions are in abeyance in the state of hypnosis, suggestions are notoriously easily implanted, and this is simply another example of the same process.

We may next consider certain other factors which modify a man's suggestibility. Those arising in the course of his contact with life are the low vitality induced by fatigue and sickness, the disturbances produced by emotional experiences, and the influence of the community. The factors relating to the suggested material are the source from which the suggestion is given, the manner in which it is given, and the circumstances under which it is given.

The low vitality produced by fatigue and illness is a potent factor in increasing suggestibility and falls within the experience of every one. The reason of this is that when our vitality is low, we feel physically feeble and incapable of acting for ourselves, and so our self-reliance is diminished and our abasement gains ascendancy over our self-assertion. In addition, being fatigued, we find we have not our usual power of marshalling our knowledge ; we do not actually lose anything out of our store of known facts, but we cannot find the requisite ones quickly, and so our power of reasoning and of making quick decisions is lessened. This interferes with our power of criticizing suggestions, and makes us more liable to follow them, since this is the line of least resistance.

A tendency to negativism, to do exactly the opposite to what is suggested, is sometimes met with in sick people and in children. McDougall has shown that this is likely to be well developed in persons with a strong tendency to self-assertion, and it originates either from a dislike for the person who is trying to suggest things or from the unwise method which he employs to instil the suggestion. It is, for example, often seen in sick people, when the attendant has been over-fussy in trying to make the patient do something for which he is not inclined. This exception, however, does not interfere with the general rule, that low vitality tends to increase suggestibility.

In states of extreme emotional disturbance suggestibility is increased, and the more intense the emotional feeling the greater is the suggestibility. As Drever [1] has pointed out, the intensity of emotional feeling increases with the resistance to the realization of the normal activity, which the individual should exhibit as a result of the emotion. Hence a man who is in a situation where a powerful emotion, such as fear or anger, is aroused, but where the normal activities of flight or attack are impossible, tends to be very highly suggestible. The reason for this is that in intense emotion it is only the affective patterns which achieve consciousness, while principles, reason, logic, and all higher thought activities are outside the field of attention. Hence a suggestion coming from the outside finds no organized resistance to its activities and has a greater chance to activate associated action patterns.

The influence of a person's social community has a great power of increasing the suggestibility of the individual. Man is a gregarious animal, and all his ideas and actions are influenced by the dictates of his herd. People for the most part hold convictions and regulate their behaviour, not by the light of reason, but because their ' set ' thinks and acts like that, and to think or act differently is ' bad form.' Even in the case of social rebels, who would appear to be exceptions to this rule, it is generally found that they are members of a small clique, within the greater herd, and that they adhere even more closely to the dictates of the small coterie than do the members of the larger community to their code of social ethics. There can be no doubt that the very fact of being

---

[1] J. Drever, *Instinct in Man.* Cambridge 1917.

L

suggestible to the dictates of his immediate associates renders
the individual less suggestible to influences coming from outside the herd, but this does not alter the fact, that the more
closely an individual is bound up in a community, the more
suggestible he becomes. The factor underlying this suggestibility is the feeling of self-abasement in the individual in
face of the composite force of the whole community, and the
fact that he is frequently forced to accept situations, in which
his individual reasoning powers are not allowed to act. This
suggestibility is well seen in the behaviour of crowds, more
particularly when the suggestibility is increased by the
presence of intense emotions. Hence an orator is able to
sway a crowd to his will, if he first arouses the emotions of its
members and then instils suggestions. It is to be noted,
however, that he must be, or pretend to be, in sympathy
with the general opinion of the crowd to begin with, so that
he appears to be speaking from within the herd, otherwise
he will tend to arouse opposition rather than compliance.

The factors relating to the suggestion which increase
suggestibility can be dismissed shortly. The source of the
suggestion is more effective the greater the prestige it possesses,
since such prestige leads to self-abasement. Thus, if the suggestion is given by one person to another, the greater the
authority that person has, whether by reason of his rank
or peculiar knowledge of the subject, the stronger will be the
suggestion.

We must next examine the circumstances under which
hysterical symptoms are produced. Two factors must be
clearly distinguished in this respect. The first is the psychical
factor which increases the subject's suggestibility, and the
second is the physical factor which determines the nature of the
hysterical symptom, for, according to the theory of hysteria
here upheld, the hysterical symptom is always due to the
perpetuation or exaggeration of a physical disturbance in the

personality at the time when the suggestibility was increased. It would seem that hysterical symptoms may be produced under six sets of circumstances, and in each of these it is necessary to define the psychical influence, which increases the suggestibility, and the physical influence, which determines the nature of the symptom. Probably in all cases both factors operate to a certain extent, but their relative preponderance varies enormously, for in some cases the psychical factor, by markedly increasing the suggestibility of the patient, allows a relatively slight physical suggestion to be perpetuated as an hysterical symptom, while in other cases the physical suggestion is so strong that the symptom will be impressed on a person of relatively low suggestibility. It is convenient to arrange the groups of hysterical symptoms in such an order, as will represent descending grades of psychical suggestibility.

The first group is found in those people who have acquired a sense of inferiority either in respect of their whole body or of one or more limbs or organs. For such patients, who are hypochondriacal in their expectation of illness, the slightest physical accident, or passing ache or pain is sufficient to determine an hysterical symptom either affecting the whole body or the particular limb or organ, which is believed to be weak. Such people are obviously ill-adjusted to themselves and towards life, and their suggestibility is markedly pathological. It is increased by the patients' general pattern of self-abasement and by their conflicts and the consequent decrease in the powers of integration and discrimination. These prevent them using their reasoning and critical powers to full advantage, and so they are unable to examine the value of the physical cause of their hysterical symptoms. Further, as their condition progresses, they get really ill and their vitality is lowered, and so they become more suggestible, while the emotion of self-pity which is aroused works still further in the same direction. In such cases, the hysterical symptom may be of any variety, as the slightest physical stimulus will be responded to.

In the next group, the hysterical symptoms are sequels of commotion. Here some actual physical trauma, such as a blow on the head, has, without necessarily causing complete loss of consciousness, led to general confusion of the patient's mind. This may lead to a very temporary inability to hear or to see or remember. Under such circumstances, the patient's suggestibility is increased by the complete abolition of the power of reasoning and criticizing. His active consciousness is temporarily in abeyance and impressions are made under conditions, in which he is more than usually amenable to suggestion. Under such circumstances, the fact that he cannot hear, see, or remember, suggests to him that he must be deaf, blind, or have lost his memory. Having received this suggestion he ceases to listen, to look, or to try to remember, so that, until he is treated, he is hysterically deaf, blind, or amnesic. These three hysterical symptoms have been quoted because they are the most characteristic of this group, but paralysis, dumbness, and other manifestations may result under the same circumstances.

The third group consists of symptoms produced under stress of great emotion. In such cases, if the natural outlet of the emotion is blocked, the intensity of the effect increases, and with this, the extent of the physical expressions of emotion. These latter are useful in their incipient stages, but become useless, if they are intensified by the deflection of all the energy which ought to be used in the performance of the normal active sequel of the emotion. Symptoms induced in this way include dumbness and stammering, rigidity, tremor and collapse of the legs, and excessive purposeless movements ; these physical phenomena are perpetuated as hysterical mutism, stammering, tremor, and paraplegia, and, in the case of the purposeless movements, as hysterical tics or fits. The increased suggestibility is determined by the complete dominance of the active consciousness by the emotion and consequent loss of reasoning powers. In the case of fear, under the stress of which hysterical symptoms are specially prone to develop, there is definite self-abasement in the presence of some overwhelming situation. In the case of panics or mob anger, the suggestibility may also be increased by the influence of the herd, as was discussed above, but this would be in a general rather than in a particular way.

The next group consists of symptoms produced by heterosuggestion. These are generally the result of some unwise remark or action on the part of the physician or nurse, which conveys to the patient the suggestion that he has some physical disability. Several psychical factors come into play. Firstly, there is the self-abasement which the patient feels in the presence of the physician, especially in respect of his knowledge of the subject, and his own lack of organized knowledge will itself prevent proper criticism of the suggestion. Then we have objective factors in the prestige of the physician, the manner in which he makes the remark, and the circumstances under which it is made. For example, a distinguished physician remarked in the presence of an assembly of other physicians, all apparently agreeing, that the patient had a disease which would result in paralysis of both legs. The suggestion was accepted, and paraplegia, although the diagnosis was quite wrong, ultimately developed. Or again, if a physician very carefully and with considerable ceremony examines for anæsthesia, asking if the patient feels this and this, the patient thinks he is expected to have anæsthesia and will readily develop it.

The fifth group comprises those symptoms acquired by imitation from another patient. The physical stimulus is here more defined, and symptoms are acquired, such as stammering, abnormal movements, and various gaits seen in other patients. The psychical stimulus, in this case, is due to self-abasement felt by the imitator in face of another person, whom he regards as very wonderful or very extraordinary, and to a certain interference with the critical powers, induced by the emotion of curiosity and the influence of the herd. Here, however, the psychical element is of much less importance, for the tendency to imitate is strong in us all and it does not require much suggestibility to determine the perpetuation of the imitated symptom, which quickly becomes a habit. Such imitated symptoms are not as a rule severe, but may be remarkably persistent.

The last group comprises symptoms which are habit continuations of definite but temporary organic disabilities, which may range from blindness and deafness, through vomiting and urinary troubles, to paralysis, contractures and anæsthesia. Here the physical stimulus is enormously strong, for it actually is present in the patient's own body. The psychical factor of increased suggestibility is present to a slighter degree and may be induced by low vitality, owing to the illness and to the difficulty experienced by the patient in adjusting himself to life.

The conclusions which one would wish to draw are :

(1) There is nothing necessarily pathological about suggestibility, which is an innate tendency present in every individual.

(2) That hysterical symptoms are met with in patients who are obviously pathologically suggestible, in which case they are the least important, though they may be the most obvious part of the disease ; but

(3) Hysterical symptoms are very commonly met with in individuals, who are not so obviously pathologically suggestible under ordinary circumstances.

(4) Hysterical symptoms are induced in such individuals

by a temporary increase in the suggestibility, due to environmental or endopsychic causes ; but

(5) Where the suggestion is strong enough, this temporary increase of suggestibility may be so slight as to be practically negligible, and when the hysterical symptom is removed, the patient is as normal as his neighbour.

The fundamental difference between this consideration of hysteria as a direct result of suggestion, and that adopted by the followers of Charcot and the German schools is, that in our conception of hysteria, we regard the condition as a superimposition on a more or less severe neurosis and do not label the patient hysterical unless hysterical symptoms are actually manifested.

In examining a case in which any physical disability whatever is present, hysteria should always be kept in mind. It is a truism to say that every disease has its functional element, and this is often much larger than is at first expected. For example, Hurst describes a case of hemiplegia admitted to hospital for observation. On examination he presented contractures of the arm and leg and marked facial paralysis. His reflexes were those usually associated with pyramidal lesions. The condition had come on in the course of an attack of arthritis. To all appearances he was a hopeless case. He was treated, however, as if he was an obviously hysterical case, and to the surprise of everybody he improved in the most remarkable way. Eventually he went home, after about six weeks' stay in hospital, suffering from a slight limp, able to do fine work with his affected hand, and with no facial paralysis. His reflexes were still the same as on admission, showing a slight residual affection of his pyramidal tract. This of course was a very marked example of the occurrence of a functional element superimposed on an organic condition, but some degree of such functional disability is certainly present in every malady.

In this connexion it used to be taught, that the first thing to do was to remove the organic element so far as possible, and then deal with the hysterical part. Experience has shown, however, that the long time and special measures necessary in dealing with an organic disability simply impress the idea of illness more firmly on the patient's mind. He is, therefore, subjected to a stronger suggestion, and the counter-suggestion and persuasion necessary to remove the functional part will have a greater obstacle to contend against. Therefore, in dealing with a case, whatever its nature, the first question that the physician must ask himself is : " Can the whole of the existing disability be adequately explained by the obvious organic changes which have taken place ? " If not, any disability not depending on organic change should be regarded as hysterical and treated accordingly. The second question he should ask himself is : " Is there any chance of my harming the patient in the course of the manipulations I may have to employ to remove the functional element ? " In other words, he has got to eliminate the presence of a tuberculous or an acutely inflamed joint, such conditions as a pachymeningitis or an acute infection of any kind. He should be able to do this in a very short examination and having satisfied himself that no condition exists in which he can do harm, he should at once proceed with his psychotherapy and leave more detailed and elaborate examination until after the functional element in the condition has been removed. For just as elaborate and long treatment fixes the idea of illness, so does elaborate and long examination.

As an example of this, one has only got to remember the number of cases of hysterical aphonia, which were perpetuated during the war by the careful but unfortunate laryngoscopic examination of the too scientific specialist.

It was undoubtedly true that during the war many hysterical symptoms were very easily cured by methods of simple suggestion or persuasion, and that they remained cured without any elaborate psychological investigation and with no signs of mental abnormality of any sort. In these cases the failure of adaptation was temporary and incident at the time of onset of the symptoms, but, by the time the latter were removed, the difficulty in adaptation had passed away. Moreover, in the majority of these patients the difficulty was between the ego as a whole and his environment. It is necessary, however, in all cases to give the patient an explanation of the cause which will save his self-respect, otherwise he feels that he is being accused of malingering, a charge which he knows to be unjust. This may lead him to cling to his symptom to save himself from being despised both by others and by himself.

In peace-time practice, on the other hand, it is the universal experience that hysterical symptoms of the patient are generally much more difficult to remove than those which were met with during the war, and when removed, the patient still exhibits an abnormal mental condition. This is because in these cases the failure of adaptation is within the ego, between opposing patterns in his make-up, and these, as a rule, cannot be reconciled and integrated, without some psychotherapeutic assistance. Moreover, in so far as the hysterical symptom may serve as a compromise of sorts in the conflict, unsatisfactory as this may be, its removal may intensify the mental symptoms instead of relieving them, as happens in the former case.

As will be seen by reference to Chapter XV, where this aspect of suggestion is considered, suggestion can only act when it is associated in some way with a pattern already established within the patient's personality. As an example of the first variety of hysterical symptom we may quote the case of a young man, who, while a prisoner of war in Germany, had his knuckles bruised by a heavy piece of metal falling across his hand. The suggestion arising from the pain, resulted in an hysterical paralysis of the flexor muscles so that the fingers were held rigidly extended. This condition lasted nine months, till he came home after the war and was brought to hospital. Here he was found not only to be suffering from the paralysis of his fingers, but also from considerable anxiety lest he should prove unable to earn his living in civil life. Five minutes' explanation and persuasion "cured" his paralysis and his anxiety. In this case he had certainly found it difficult to adapt to the conditions of prison life in Germany, which pertained at the onset, but these difficult conditions had entirely passed away at the time of cure. There was no significant conflict within the ego but only between the ego and the environment.

An example of the second class is afforded by a lady who was the victim of an intense and complicated conflict between her ego ideal and her more primitive impulses, with the result that an obsession of suicide supervened, the idea of which was strongly opposed by her sense of morality. One day she stumbled over a low parapet, fell on her back, and from the suggestion of spinal injury acquired an hysterical paralysis of her lower limbs. This was a good example of the compromise symptom, since she remarked with some satisfaction: "Now I can't throw myself out of the window, even if I wanted to."

It is to be noticed that in both these cases the symptom served a purpose, in the first place achieving an amelioration of conditions and in the second setting up a barrier against suicide. Lately Kretschmer [1] has drawn further attention to this purposeful nature of hysterical symptoms and also to the fact that many symptoms are in accordance with instinctive reactions, and that these two factors seem to reinforce each other in many instances.

Let us examine the nature of the reactions quoted in greater detail. The young soldier as a prisoner of war was being forced

[1] E. Kretschmer, *Hysteria* (Nervous and Mental Diseases. Monograph, Ser. 44). New York 1926.

to work against his will, under circumstances of considerable emotional stress and unpleasant affect—fear, anxiety and even hunger and want of sleep. Such emotional stress is apt to result in regression, that is the exhibition of patterns of behaviour characteristic of a lower level of development than that appropriate to his age and circumstances. Consider the reaction of the child being forced to do something he does not want—how he tightens up all his muscles in a violent effort of protest and resistance. Under the circumstances of the prisoners' camp, although our young man was not actually behaving in this way, he was emotionally and mentally set, so that it would not have taken much to induce that pattern of rigid resistance. One day a heavy bar falls on his knuckles and pain inhibits the action of the flexor muscles, so that the hand is held rigidly still, a pattern all the more readily adopted in view of the set referred to above. So far as the hand is concerned, therefore, this pattern of rigidity is doubly determined and the inhibition of flexor activity becomes more or less permanent, since it suits the most insistent influence in his personality, namely the desire to avoid work under extremely adverse circumstances. In other words, rigidity of the fingers becomes part of a more general and more influential pattern. This process of conditioning so that a subsidiary pattern becomes part of a more generalized pattern is quite a commonplace all through individual development, and on it depends a great deal of learning by experience. For example, the chick who pecks at all bright objects is inhibited from pecking at the bitter red ladybird, after experience, and thereafter this avoidance of ladybirds becomes part of his " pecking pattern." This case illustrates another interesting and difficult psychological problem. In Germany the general " go " of the personality was to avoid work. The subjective pattern or complex, related to work (W), was therefore in repulsion as regards a job (J), and when the pattern of immobility of hand (IH) was incorporated, there was no endopsychic disharmony, *i.e.*, no anxiety, thus :

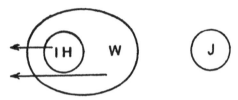

But in England the general go of the personality was to get and do work, and therefore (W) was in appetition as regards (J), but now the incorporated pattern (IH) was still in repulsion thus :

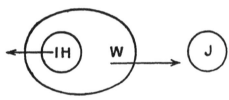

and so here we have endopsychic disharmony and conflict and consequently anxiety.   In order to restore harmony and abolish anxiety we have to remove or destroy (IH), and in the case quoted, when this was done, cure resulted.   On the other hand, while the war was still on, it often happened that removal of an hysterical symptom, such as paralysis of an arm, induced anxiety, where none was present before.   The usual situation in war which could not be met was roughly that ideals pattern (I) induced appetition towards war (W), while self-preservation patterns (SP) urged repulsion in respect to war thus :

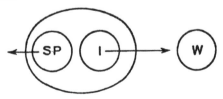

Result endopsychic conflict and anxiety. Then suggestion from a minor injury induced hysterical paralysis (P), regarded as inevitable by the subject, hence (I) was satisfied and appetition was neutralized, so that retirement from war was possible and endopsychic conflict and anxiety was abolished, thus :

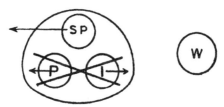

But if war was still going on and we destroy P, conflict is re-established and anxiety returns. Though this process is less common in times of peace, it is still to be met with in hysterical cases in association with the workmen's compensation and pensions acts.

Of a similar nature is our second example. Without going into the complexities of the case we have difficulty of facing life due to varying causes. From this we have a conflict —desire to escape all obligations—suicide (S) versus—a desire to play the game and to live in accordance with very strong and real religious convictions (R) thus :

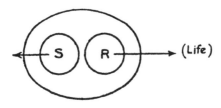

Hence conflict and anxiety. Then comes a minor accident, firmly believed to be a major accident, resulting in paralysis

(P), and therefore not in conflict with religious scruples (R), but making suicide impossible, thus :

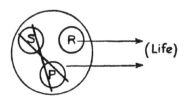

For the time being conflict is relieved and anxiety disappears or is decreased. Later, however, paralysis (P) comes into conflict with religious scruples (R), because it is a useless, selfish life, to lie doing nothing and being waited on by others. The degree to which this secondary conflict will arise will depend on the absolute or partial success of the suggestion. If the patient had been absolutely convinced of the inevitability and permanence of the paralysis no conflict would arise, but, if there was still some doubt as to its nature, this secondary conflict would develop sooner or later.

How a subsidiary incorporated pattern is detached from the more general pattern as is bound to occur in the dissociation which determines the production of an hysterical symptom, is a matter of great interest and extreme importance in the study of the neurotic. This detachment of a subsidiary pattern from one main pattern and its reattachment to another is a constant feature, both in the induction and cure of neurosis, and, although it applies in relation to hysteria, its most obviously important application is to obsessions, and the problem has been discussed in this connexion in Chapter VI.

The subject of hysteria cannot be left without further discussion of Freud's theory of the nature of hysterical symptoms. We must confine ourselves here to that variety of Freud's much wider conception of hysteria, which he calls conversion hysteria. The symptoms of conversion hysteria are, according to him, symbolic of repressed wishes, and are specially liable to occur in those parts of the body which are the seat of what Adler afterwards called organ inferiority. Ernest Jones [1] refers to this as follows : " He finds that there is frequently a special predisposition of a given part of the body to discharge the energy that is flowing in an aberrant path. The choice of a particular symptom is thus determined, not entirely by the mental associations or symbolisms present, but also by the attraction that a given sensitive part of the body, which is perhaps defective or actually diseased, may present towards any symbolic process that is possible." The importance of this organ inferiority in the determination of hysterical symptoms has already been discussed, it remains to investigate whether symbolization of repressed wishes is really antagonistic to the theory here expounded, that symptoms are due to suggestion at the time of onset. In Chapter XV suggestion is discussed, and it is shown that the suggested idea does nothing of itself, but merely serves as a stimulus to the activation of a pattern already in existence in the personality. Let us take a case of hysterical blindness with blepharospasm. An ordinary anamnesis of the case disclosed the fact that the blindness came on after a painful attack of conjunctivitis. Here was the suggestion which determined the blepharospasm and blindness, but in this case ordinary persuasion and suggestion did not effect a cure and a deeper analysis of the condition was undertaken. To cut a long story short—though this process of curtailing such stories detracts from the credibility of the clinical reports,—the patient himself gave an indication of the trouble, when he said he could not bear to look himself in the face. This was because he felt great remorse in respect of certain habits. He was brought to regard these things more normally and with a better sense of proportion, and after the symbolic connexion was pointed out

---

[1] E. Jones, *Treatment of the Neuroses.* London 1920.

to him, a very little persuasion removed his blindness. In this case, which has been considerably simplified for the purpose of illustrating the point at issue, the suggestion—the attack of conjunctivitis—simply acted as a stimulus to determine the activation of a pattern involving unwillingness to face and look at a situation, which was symbolically expressed by actually closing the eyes and ceasing to look. It follows then, that in many cases the suggestion will determine a symbolic expression of some conative pattern within the personality, but it does not follow that every hysterical symptom is necessarily a symbol of some deep-lying complex, or that it needs an elaborate analysis to cure it. Inexperienced analysts are sometimes singularly blind to this and strive to find complicated explanations where no complex situation exists. This ought to be avoided both in regard to the reputation of the physician and to the patience and purse of the hysterical subject. Such then is the general conception of the nature of hysteria ; it remains to examine the various types of hysterical symptom which may occur.

CHAPTER IX

HYSTERICAL SYMPTOMS

A BRIEF review of the symptoms which may be described as hysterical seems to be desirable, in order to illustrate the thesis here put forward, both in respect of neurosis in general and hysteria in particular. A complete discussion of each would obviously be redundant so that most have been merely described, but the physiological and psychological points of view have been dealt with in the case of tremors and fits, which seem to lend themselves to such discussion.

Hysterical Paralysis.—This subject has been so much discussed in medical literature and its occurrence is so familiar to the majority of physicians, that prolonged description is not necessary here.

Paralyses may be either flaccid or spastic, and in certain cases a mixed type is met with. The flaccid type simulates a lesion of the lower motor neurone and may follow such organic conditions of a temporary character. The spastic type simulates lesions of the cortico-pyramidal tract and the distinction is often difficult, but in most hysterical cases there will be no interference with the deep tendon reflexes, which are outside voluntary control.

It is important to notice certain points of differentiation between organic and functional paralyses and to consider their diagnostic value.

(1) Abdominal reflexes are absent in pyramidal lesions, but normally can only be elicited if the abdominal muscles

M   177

are relaxed. This relaxation is often hard to obtain in hysterical subjects, so this sign is of no certain value.

(2) The knee jerks are exaggerated in pyramidal lesions. In hysterical cases the muscles are sometimes so rigid that the reflexes cannot be obtained at all, but at other times they are apparently much exaggerated. A useful distinction, however, is the following : If the reflex is tested by tapping the patella or tibia instead of the tendon, in pyramidal lesions the knee jerk will be readily obtained off the bone, but this is not usually so in functional cases.

(3) Ankle jerks are, as a rule, unaffected in hysterical cases, and exaggerated in pyramidal lesions, but it is difficult to set up any standard for comparison.

(4) Ankle and patellar clonus is present in pyramidal lesions, but is very frequently present in hysterical cases also, for any attempt to move a spastic limb produces clonic movements. As a rule, in hysterical cases, they are less regular than is the case in organic lesions, but sometimes no distinction can be made.

(5) Plantar reflexes. In pyramidal lesions there is dorsiflexion of the big toe, and fanning of the rest, but this is not present in hysterical cases, unless it may be produced by the suggestion of the examining physician. This latter condition is certainly rare, but has been met with. It is important to notice that in many hysterical cases, disuse has interfered with the blood supply of the limb to such an extent, that the foot is permanently cold and the reflex very difficult to elicit.

The sign of flexion of the thigh on the trunk, sometimes called Babinski's second sign, is a most useful distinction. To elicit this, the patient is laid flat on his back, with his legs stretched widely apart. He is then told to clasp his arms on his chest and rise to the sitting posture. In pyramidal lesions the paralysed leg rises into the air. In hysterical cases, either the legs do not move off the ground or the sound leg rises.

While discussing differential signs of organic and hysterical paralysis, certain less important distinctions between the two which have been described from time to time in the literature, may be mentioned. In facial paralysis the platysma sign, that is, paralysis of the platysma on the affected side has been supposed to be significant of organic origin, but this is definitely not the case, for the platysma has been observed to be paralysed in many hysterical patients. In paralysis of the arms, tossing the pronated forearms into the air has been described as a pathognomonic distinction. The organic cases fall in a position of supination and the hysterical cases in pronation. In some cases of unilateral pyramidal lesions, strong movements of the healthy limb produce corresponding automatic movements in the affected limb. This does not occur in hysterical cases. In many cases of extensive hysterical paralysis there is an anæsthesia of the limb involved, because paralysis is usually associated with anæsthesia in the mind of the patient. This, however, cannot be regarded as a sign of much importance.

To distinguish between organic and hysterical paralysis, the observer must have a clear idea of what he expects to find in a pyramidal lesion or in a lesion involving the anterior cells or peripheral nerves, for if there is any discrepancy in the reflex findings, or in the muscles involved, hysteria must be presumed. In this connexion, however, it is of the utmost importance to realize that, where there has been a temporary organic derangement, function will be restored long before the reflex changes return to normal. A familiar example occurs in diphtheritic paralysis, in which the tendon reflexes are absent long after the child can walk again. Less familiar to all, though of course recognized by neurologists, is the fact that after pyramidal lesions, function may be restored, while the plantar reflex is still dorsiflexor, and while exaggerated tendon reflexes are still present. In such cases the paralysis may continue as an hysterical symptom, and the observer is misled by all the signs of organic disease being present. A case illustrating this has already been described. It is a very good rule to approach a case of paralysis with the possibility of hysteria uppermost in the mind of the observer, for no harm is done if it turns out to be organic, but many a chance of rapid recovery is missed by a too hasty conclusion as to the organic nature of the disability.

Hysterical paralysis is frequently accompanied by contractures. These follow immobility of a part however produced ; most frequently they occur as the result of pain, which forbids the movement of the affected part, but the immobility persists after pain has ceased. In such cases, secondary pain is often induced, resulting from muscular spasms, malpositions of the limbs and abnormal pressures on joints. This pain is relieved when the contracture is relaxed.

A common origin of contracture is the immobilization of a limb by splints, the position persisting after the splint has been removed. No good object can be attained by describing the various forms of contracture and their resultant postures, for any position, which can be voluntarily assumed, or produced by mechanical device, may be maintained as an hysterical contracture, and can be diagnosed easily by careful observation as to whether the actual injury could have caused the disability or not. It is important, in this connexion, to mention the reflex disorders described by Babinski and Froment [1] as the results of war injuries. The researches of Hurst,[2] Reeves, and others in this country, and of Roussy and others in France, have conclusively proved

[1] Babinski and Froment, *Hysterie-Pithiatisme.* Paris 1917.
[2] A. F. Hurst, *War Contractures (Brit. Journ. of Surg.,* 1918).

that these are all hysterical, the result of suggestion and curable by psychotherapy. The various trophic and vascular changes, though not themselves hysterical, are nevertheless dependent on the immobility and want of use of the part, which results from the hysterical paralysis. These secondary symptoms themselves disappear when the paralysis is cured and movement and function are restored. They consist of coldness and numbness of the part, lessening of the amplitude of the pulse, stiffness and loss of elasticity of the ligaments and fibrous tissue, trophic changes in the skin and nails, shrinking in the size of muscles and subcutaneous tissues, with alteration in their electrical excitability and finally decalcification and rarefaction of bones as shown by X-ray photographs. The important point is to realize that these secondary signs do not exclude hysteria as a diagnosis, but are dependent simply on immobility and disuse.

While localized paralyses are generally the sequels of temporary organic lesions, the more generalized cases frequently follow intense emotional shock with a resultant loss of control of the limbs. This implants a suggestion of inability to move, which may persist as an hysterical symptom.

The actual symptom complex is the result of a dissociation of a pattern involving certain neurones. The nature of the symptom will depend on the level at which the inhibition takes place. It is sometimes said that hysterical symptoms depend on interference with function at cortical levels, and organic symptoms may depend on interference with function at any level of the nervous system, but this will not bear examination, if we refer to the locality of the inhibition. Experiments and clinical observation show that muscles and muscle groups are represented in the spinal cord, but that movements are represented on the cortex. That is to say, that if we destroy motor cells in the spinal cord, certain muscles will be paralysed, and a given movement will only be impossible if no other muscles can bring about this movement. On the other hand if we destroy motor cells in the cortex, movements become impossible quite independently of the muscles which bring them about.   Hysterical paralyses fall into three groups :

(1) Local paralysis of muscles usually following a temporary injury of spinal motor cells. In such cases, although the motor cells have recovered the power of function, they are still inhibited, and muscular action does not take place. This is determined by suggestion, and will certainly be more resistant to being overcome, if the resultant paralysis is of any use to the patient, or to any of the patterns into which his personality has become more or less dissociated. Such an example was cited in the last chapter. The word " suggestibility " cannot explain just why the cells which were injured should remain inhibited, though it no doubt determines the " form " of the pattern, which eventually becomes inhibited. This inhibited pattern must become involved in a larger pattern involving emotional dispositions, for it is within such patterns, under pleasure and pain and affective reactions, that inhibitions and facilitations occur. What causes an inhibition or facilitation we do not know, but analogy with pharmacological action brings strong presumptive evidence that the process is a biochemical one. It is the affective reaction, with the activation of the vegetative and endocrine systems which sets up these biochemical changes. For this reason, even in respect of the most obvious results of suggestion, Hurst's contention that no mental or emotional factor lies behind such symptoms must be inadequate.

(2) The paralysis of a movement, subsequent to temporary injury to cortical motor cells is the second type of hysterical paralysis. With the exception that the distribution of the paralysis is different and that it is spastic in type instead of flaccid, there is no essential difference in the process of develop-

ment of the inhibition from that already described. On the other hand this type merges into the third variety.

(3) Paralysis involving one or more limbs as a whole, the result of emotional disturbance suggesting inability to move such parts of the body is the third type. This is frequently accompanied by a corresponding anæsthesia, since paralysis and loss of sensation are so often associated in the perceptive pattern (Gestalt) of the limb. Here we have a wider range in the inhibition, involving cortical cells outside the motor area and still more intimately connected with the larger dissociated emotional patterns, so that clinically the underlying mental factor is at once more obvious and important.

Tremors.—The occurrence of tremors and inco-ordinations as physical symptoms amongst neurotic patients is so common, that they have often been passed by as too obvious to require comment. Sometimes, however, the careful investigation of such obvious symptoms throws light on more obscure problems, and as the general pathology of tremor has been worked out fairly fully it seems to present an opportunity for a full examination of the connexion between an hysterical and an organic symptom. The subject of neurotic tremor has received a good deal of attention from the French. Roussy and Lhermitte [1] describe two varieties, atypical and typical. The former they regard as expressions of the emotion of fear, and Meige [2] has pointed out that in extreme cases they may form part of an obsession characterized by a phobia of tremor, in which the greater the phobia the more intense the tremor. The latter variety of tremors, which resemble those typical of various organic nervous diseases, are regarded as imitative. During the war, Meige gave a bad prognosis as to their cura-

[1] Roussy and Lhermitte, *The Psychoneuroses of War*, p. 55 (Military Med. Manuals). London 1918.
[2] H. Meige, *Les Tremblements consécutifs aux explosions* (*Rev. Neur·*, 1916), p. 201.

bility, and argued therefrom that they were due to definite organic changes within the central nervous system. Roussy and Hurst,[1] however, deny the former contention and discredit the latter, because of the possibility of cure by psychotherapy.

Janet [2] describes hysterical inco-ordinated movements under three heads : expressive movements which include gesticulations which would properly belong to some emotional experience ; " professional " movements, such as those of reiterated piano-playing or drum-beating, and imitative movements which may be of any variety. He points out that all these tremors involve the more or less co-ordinated functions of several groups of muscles and never of single muscles, and therefore that the disturbance is at a high level of the nervous system. Further, he points out that the patients are quite conscious of these movements, but seem to have lost the feeling of liberty and volition with regard to them. Déjérine and Gauckler [3] note the variety of types of tremor, but consider that they are of emotional origin as evidenced by the fact that emotional crises will initiate or exaggerate them. They suggest that they may be phobic in origin and represent a persistent recoil from an action which is constantly being attempted. In other cases they suggest that the tremor is a constant effort to correct a vicious attitude.

Amongst English authors who have considered the subject, Hurst suggests that the tremor is always due to inco-ordinated hypertonus of antagonistic muscles, and attributes this to the suggestive effect of emotional states. Mott [4] regarded tremors as " due to defective innervation and an involuntary spread

---

[1] A. F. Hurst, *Tremor in Soldiers* (*Seale Hayne Neurological Studies*), p. 53. Oxford 1918.

[2] P. Janet, *Les Nevroses*, p. 89. Paris 1919.

[3] Déjérine and Gauckler, *Les Manifestations Fonctionelles des Psychonevroses*, p. 193. Paris 1911.

[4] F. W. Mott, *War Neuroses and Shell-shock*, p. 158. Oxford 1919.

of nervous impulses to antagonistic groups of muscles," and considered this defect of "high central origin." The originating factor is the suggestion conveyed by fear and possibly by cold. He considers that the fine tremor similar to that of chronic alcoholism, Graves' disease and general paralysis is due to fatigue, while the coarser tremors are due to suggestion and imitation. Personal investigations into the genesis of neurotic tremor have revealed a variety of pathogenic factors, but the initial influence is emotional and the particular emotion involved would seem to be fear. In my experience hysterical tremors which present themselves for treatment may be grouped under two heads. The first group consists of those which persist for a certain time as neural habits with little or no emotional accompaniment, except that induced by the tremor itself. These were common enough in the war, and are met with in civil life to a less extent. In such cases a condition of simultaneous hypertonus of antagonistic muscles is revealed, and treatment consists in teaching the patient to relax these and re-establish the proper reciprocal tonic action. Such hypertonicity and tremor are most often sequels to a painful wound or other pathological condition in the limb, which induces a fear of movement, but as soon as the painful condition has passed away, the emotional accompaniment also disappears, except in so far as some anxiety exists in view of the uselessness of the trembling limb. The removal of the tremor will be sufficient to cure the condition, since there is no abnormal emotional reaction behind it. The second group comprises those cases in which there is a definite mental accompaniment of fear or anxiety. The extent to which this affective accompaniment is conscious varies. There may be a consciousness of the object of the emotion, or of an object, though on investigation it is found that this is not the true one. In other cases there is no apparent object but simply abstract panic. Sometimes the fear is associated with and conditioned by some other emotional disposition, which may modify the localization and character of the tremor. Thus, a case of tremor of the right hand was found to be associated with fear of masturbation and its imagined results, and the nature of the object of the fear undoubtedly modified the character of the tremor. Similarly, when the organic inferiority of a limb engenders various fears and anxieties in respect of it, a definite localization and modification of the tremor may occur. With regard to the so-called imitative tremors, the nature and distribution of these may be determined by the source of the imitation, but there seems little doubt that these imitative symptoms are only initiated when the patient is already in a state of anxiety and fear. The physiological connexion of tremor with the emotion of fear may be understood if we may digress for a moment to consider the pattern which underlies it.

The emotion of fear is a primary affective disposition which is a purposive reaction to certain stimuli. The purpose is a very definite one and a very important one, namely to protect the animal against dangers to health and life. In its simplest form, the stimuli which initiate the response may be of great variety, and any noxious influence at all is capable of setting off the reaction. With increasing integration, the stimuli become more specific as the individual neglects certain of these, which he has learnt by experience to be innocuous. This learning by experience to discard certain stimuli is a process of conditioning, comparable to the classical experiments of Pawlow, but we may express the process as a negative rather than as a positive conditioning. At first any noisy object approaching sets off the fear response in a young horse in a field, but after repeated experience that the motors passing along the road beside him do not cause him any hurt, the reaction is so conditioned that he no longer responds to this particular stimulus. This discrimination is a cortical function for, as Bianchi [1] has shown, when monkeys who have learnt to discriminate between apparent and real noxious stimuli are subjected to ablation of their frontal lobes, they become subject to uncontrolled panic in the presence of stimuli which are usually quite inadequate to induce reaction. This shows that the localization of the primitive fear pattern is subcortical, and Head [2] has shown that those cases of thalamic syndrome, which are characterized by uncontrolled reactions to painful stimuli also act in an uncontrolled manner in response to other affective stimuli. We may justly presume therefore, that the localization of the principal integration of the primitive response to noxious stimuli is in the thalamus. This response involves a special differentiation of painful affect which we recognize as panic, or, if of weaker intensity and more prolonged, as anxiety. The motor response will vary according to the species of animal, and in the case of higher animals and man according to circumstances. Rivers [3] distinguishes five modes of reaction: flight, aggression, manipulative activity, immobility and collapse. With the exception of the last any power of discrimination between these various types of reaction depends on cortical function and is not part of the primary response. In addition to these responses, there are certain involuntary activities, such as dilatation of the pupil, acceleration of the pulse, dilatation of the bronchi, mobilization of blood sugar and inhibition of digestive function, together with sweating and erection of hairs, the purpose of all of which is to prepare the animal for instant action. All these activities are the result of the activation of a series of neurones arranged as a specific engram. The researches of Cannon [4] and others have shown that the engram comprises

[1] L. Bianchi, *The Mechanism of the Brain and the Function of the Frontal Lobes*, p. 185. Edinburgh 1922.

[2] Sir H. Head, *Studies in Neurology*. London 1921.

[3] W. H. R. Rivers, *Instinct and the Unconscious*, p. 52. Cambridge 1920.

[4] W. B. Cannon, *Bodily Changes in Pain, Hunger, Fear, and Rage*. London 1915.

neurones of the sympathetic system in addition to those of the central nervous system, the activities of the former being reinforced by the outpouring of suprarenal secretion into the blood. The latter factors indeed determine the accompanying involuntary activities, which we designate as characteristic of fear. In addition to these strictly purposive reactions, however, unless the reaction is perfectly controlled and discriminated, certain useless activities ensue, the most characteristic of which is tremor. Perfect control and discrimination are the functions of the cortex, while, as will be seen later, tremor is essentially a subcortical reaction. The work of Sherrington [1] and later that of Wilson has shown that the engraphic activity on which the bodily changes depend, does not have as its mental correlate the full affective experience, which probably depends on higher thalamic integration. In his research on involuntary laughing and crying Wilson definitely proved that this was not accompanied by corresponding affective experience. [2] He places the centre for these bodily affective expressions in the upper pontine region and, as there is evidence that affective experience is associated with thalamic function, we may take it that the James-Lange theory is not adequate. That is to say that affective experience is not simply the mental correlate of the bodily changes, but involves a higher integration through cells in the thalamic grey matter. The primary reaction of fear then is dependent on an engram integrated at the thalamic level and exhibits the characteristic all-or-none reaction of this level. Under ordinary circumstances in man and the higher animals this primary reaction is under cortical control, whereby discrimination is possible. Tremor, therefore, will only manifest

---

[1] Sir C. Sherrington, *Integrative Action of the Nervous System*, p. 260. London 1906.

[2] S. A. K. Wilson, *Journ. of Neurology and Psychopath*, p. 299. 1924.

itself in the absence of full cortical function, and is a release phenomenon.

Our next task is to discuss the physiology of tremor. Crouzon [1] distinguishes the various types of tremor as follows :

(1) The so-called physiological tremor described by Lamarck and Pitres in forty per cent. of a thousand normal people examined. This occurs especially in intense muscular effort and when the subject strives to find a position of equilibrium. Similarly in the normal person tremor may occur under stress of emotion, especially fear, and at the onset of fever, when doubtless it may be classed as a transitory toxic tremor.

(2) Tremors associated with organic nervous disease. The intention tremor of disseminated sclerosis is not a pure rhythmical tremor, such as occurs in subthalamic lesions, when support is withdrawn from the affected limb, as Birley and Dudgeon have pointed out,[2] since it is more marked when a voluntary effort is made. This condition is a mixture of tremor and inco-ordination. In the opinion of these authorities it is due to a lesion of the cerebello-rubral fibres and certain other cerebellar connexions in addition.

Interference with the afferent tracts of the cerebello-spinal connexions are also seen in Friedreich's ataxia and in cerebellar lesions, but these also partake of inco-ordinations rather than true tremors.

The tremors of paralysis agitans and that which occurs as a sequel of encephalitis lethargica are of a more typical nature, but are slow and coarse compared to the tremors which more specially concern us. As a rule they can be controlled voluntarily to a certain extent and do not accompany voluntary movement. For these reasons, Buzzard and

---

[1] J. Crouzon, *La Pratique Neurologique*. Ed. P. Marie. Paris 1911.
[2] J. L. Birley and L. S. Dudgeon, *Brain*, XLIV, p. 150.

Greenfield [1] consider them to be due to a release of lower nervous activity by removal of control. The lesions found in those cases which have been examined, are chiefly in the cortex, in the optic thalamus and corpus striatum. The work of Wilson and others has shown that lesions in the globus pallidus will produce similar tremor. Vogt considers that the variations in the type of tremor depend on varying degrees of disintegration of the corpus striatum, but de Lisi [2] considers this explanation unsatisfactory and attributes such varieties to lesions of other structures in the midbrain. D'Antona [3] found lesions in the putamen and globus pallidus, and also in the locus niger and dentate nucleus, and concludes that the syndrome is due to removal of control of the striate system, the putamen and caudate nucleus, over the globus pallidus and lower centres. Similarly in a case of hepato-lenticular degeneration, characterized by coarse tremor in all four limbs, Hadfield [4] found marked degeneration of the putamen and globus pallidus and also of the ansa lenticularis.

The tremor of general paralysis is more typical of pure tremor and consists of a regular rhythmic movement. The lesion in this condition is general throughout the higher levels of the nervous system, but especially affects the cortical connexions.

Of a similar nature is senile tremor, and in both these conditions demonstrable changes occur in the cortical neurones. The rare hereditary tremors may be classed here as having an organic basis.·

(3) Toxic tremors. The tremor of Graves' disease is probably of this nature and, like others, owes its effect to a more or less permanent throwing out of the functions of cortical cells,

---

[1] E. F. Buzzard and J. G. Greenfield, *Brain*, XLII, p. 305.
[2] De Lisi, *Rivista di Pat. Nerv. e Ment.*, XXVII, p. 95.
[3] S. d'Antona, *Rivista di Pat. Nerv. e Ment.*, XXVII, p. 117.
[4] G. Hadfield, *Brain*, XLVI, p. 147.

though there may be no demonstrable organic change. The tremors of alcohol, lead, mercury, and that of fatigue, have a similar origin and nature.

(4) The hysterical tremors. These usually have the character of rapid regular vibrations, but may be modified by imitations of other tremors, or by special circumstances in their pathogenesis.

From this study we may see that the inco-ordinations depend on interference with the afferent side of the cerebello-nucleus ruber or prespinal arc. The intermediate coarse tremors, such as are seen in paralysis agitans, depend on interference with the next arc or more specifically with the control exercised by the striate system over the lower centres in the midbrain. Lastly, the fine tremors depend on interference with cortical control over the basal ganglia. It is of importance to notice that in all examples of the last group there is a marked loss of control of affective reactions. Patients suffering from Graves' disease, alcoholism, G.P.I. and over-fatigue are all easily moved emotionally, and the same is true in the case of the Parkinsonian, though his peculiar rigidity makes it impossible for him to express these affective states. In all these cases, we have a diminution of cortical control over basal ganglion activity, both affective and motor, and when released from control the affective thalamic centre exercises a marked influence over the corresponding striate function. Thus Coppola,[1] referring to the localizing effect of emotion on the various pathogenic influences responsible for the Parkinsonian syndrome, remarks that the exaggerated functional activity of the thalamus, resulting from the emotion of the war, was able so to influence the lenticular nucleus that it created a locus minoris resistentiæ to noxious external agencies. Further, from the evolutionary standpoint, the

[1] A. Coppola, *Rivista di Pat. Nerv. e Ment.*, XXVII, p. 116.

thalamus and the corpus striatum at one time represented the high-water mark of nervous development, and anatomically a very large body of association fibres between these centres is demonstrable.

In our estimate of the neuroses as a whole we arrived at the conclusion that there is a want of adaptation both in respect of the environment as a whole and of the particular aspects of the personality. Such adaptation essentially depends on the establishment of cortical function at its highest level and neurotic symptoms correspond to an interference with this function. These higher functions may be summarized as control, integration, discrimination and reference in time and space ; all these are noticeably deficient in the neurotic.

To return to the normal engram which subserves the fear reaction, we have seen that this is a complicated arrangement involving both the central nervous system and the sympathetic system. The function of the latter is to prepare the body in every way for instant action, in many cases flight. In the well-organized engram, which is not interfered with or conditioned by other engrams responding to simultaneous stimuli, such flight or other activity will immediately ensue. Even in normal subjects however, when this immediate action is impeded by the activity of another engram, say that subserving curiosity, there would appear to be a failure of discrimination and control and the higher cortical centres being in abeyance, there is a short circuiting at the level of the basal ganglia. One of the effects of this uncontrolled activity at this level is tremor. Under these conditions we also find both agonist and antagonist muscles held in increased postural tone ready for action, but in the absence of cortical discriminative function, neither relaxes to allow the other to act. It is suggested therefore that the muscular rigidity is rather a concomitant than a causal factor of the tremor. When cases are cured by mere re-education in relaxation of the muscles as in our first group of tremors, we are probably dealing with a condition of phobia of the tremor as described by Meige, and when the muscles are relaxed by the restoration of cortical discrimination, there is also a re-establishment of control over the striate centres, so that the tremor ceases and the phobia is removed. In the second group of tremors depending on the fear reaction, we find this is not subserved by a well-organized engram ready for prompt response, as we have seen, because of the patient's constitutional temperamental qualities, hence the cortical control is never at its best, and the establishment of the short circuiting thalamic-striate, fear-tremor response is easy and frequent.

The nature of the tremor will depend on the levels unmasked in the devolutionary process of removal of control. Where cortical control only is in abeyance, whether from the fear reactions in the anxiety states or from fatigue in the exhaustion syndrome—the most common form of hysterical tremor—there will be a fine tremor simulating the toxic tremors. When striate control is removed, there will be coarse tremors, as in the pseudo-Parkinsonian syndrome, not uncommon in hysterics. Where still lower controls, such as those of the cerebellum are removed, there will be inco-ordinations, similar to those which occur in organic interference with the afferent side of the prespinal arc.

In addition to this, tremors will be modified by the process of conditioning. For example, in the masturbatory tremor referred to above, at first two separate engrams were involved. In the first a sexual stimulus, probably ideational, set off activity in an engram which subserved certain muscular movements of the hand in contact with the genital organ, accompanied by sexual feeling and finally orgasm. Secondly, orgasm acted as a stimulus to a fear reaction, which, being poorly organized, easily became a fear-tremor syndrome. From being consecutive in their activity, these engrams became

N

coincident and the sex stimulus set off activity, which subserved a fear feeling rather than a sex feeling, and the motor
activity became a masturbatory tremor. This analysis is
superficial for the sake of clarity, for it omits the regression
to childish reaction which undoubtedly occurred.

In this way, it would seem, neurotic tremors may be
explained as to their nature, but the question, which has not
been considered is : What is the factor, either hereditary or
acquired, which is responsible for the ease with which cortical
control is inhibited and the thalamic striate short circuit
allowed to develop ? Any effort to explain this must be highly
speculative, but it is suggested that irregularity in the adrenal
secretion is the factor responsible. Inhibition is generally
held to be due to some biochemical change at the synapses,
and if we are to explain the variations in inhibitions and
facilitations, we must postulate a specific action of the biochemical inhibitive agent on certain synapses. Such specific
action is familiar in pharmacology, through the well-known
actions of such drugs as strychnine and curare on nerve endings.
In the fear reaction, it has been experimentally shown by
Cannon,[1] that there is a large output of adrenalin into the blood ;
if this is excessive, the secondary reactions of fear depending
on sympathetic activity are over-determined and uncontrolled,
and amongst these tremor is prominent. This is at least
suggestive, that excessive adrenal activity may result in
inhibition of certain cortical controls and so account for the
symptoms.

This rather elaborate analysis of tremor has been given to
show that psychic influences do modify bodily reactions at
various levels, and in a manner at least comparable to that of
organic disease.

Tics.—These are spasmodic movements of muscle groups,

[1] W. B. Cannon, *Bodily Changes in Pain, Hunger, Fear and Rage*.
London 1915.

which may be conscious or unconscious, and result in clonic jerking of the part affected. The nature of the tics has long been in dispute, and organic, psychasthenic and hysterical tics have all been described. It is suggested that very many tics are hysterical in origin, or in other words the result of suggestion. By far the commonest is the flinching tic, which is consequent upon the emotion of fear, or the tic may be an expression of aversion associated with disgust. However, all varieties are met with, and no purpose can be served by describing them at length. They are often curable, but, if they have persisted for a long time, a neural habit is established which involves a vicious circle of stimulus and response below the level of conscious control. Two examples may illustrate this : The first was a middle-aged man suffering from an apparently typical spasmodic torticollis—a rhythmic jerking of his head to one side. This tic was a very great distress to him both in his work and in his hobbies. He had been a keen golfer and his malady of course prevented him from playing at all. As is the case with many patients suffering from this disability, it was found that he was the subject of fibrositis or muscular rheumatism in the trapezius muscle on the side to which the head turned. The movement relaxed the trapezius muscle and so eased the pain of the rheumatism. A careful investigation of the history showed that the origin of the tic coincided with an acute attack of muscular rheumatism in the corresponding shoulder. Treatment of this latter condition, coupled with psychotherapy to relieve the associated anxiety, and re-education to re-establish control over the neural habit, which had been formed, succeeded in almost abolishing the tic. It was only on fatigue or agitation that the spasm was troublesome and the patient was able to resume his golf and other hobbies. In this case the suggestive influence was the chance discovery that the movement relieved pain, but the muscular response to repeated stimulus became too automatic and the control of higher cortical levels was lost.

The second case was that of a young girl sent into hospital for supposed epilepsy associated with spasmodic torticollis. Very frequently during the day her head was turned to one side and her facial muscles were contorted ; the movements were quite different from those of the man described above, and represented a gesture of aversion with an expression of disgust. From time to time she would partially lose consciousness and her whole body would be convulsed, but this was no epileptic fit, but an hysterical attack, in which all sorts of pantomimic gestures were introduced, many of which were frankly erotic. Investigation showed that there was a marked endopsychic conflict relating to a sudden and violent repression of sex in mid-adolescence. When this was cleared up the general attacks ceased entirely and the tic became much less violent and frequent. The complete cure of the latter was not effected, although all mental anxiety ceased, probably because the neural habit had become established and was no longer subject to higher control.

Fits.—Hysterical fits were very common during the war and are by no means rare under peace conditions. The onset of the fit is found to depend on an emotional crisis, and, as is the case with many neurotic symptoms, such a fit is the result of the diversion of activity, which ought to complete the action called for by the stimulus of an instinctive process. It is not by any means easy to discover in every case the psychological process, by which the suggestion was accepted, but the following examples, some of war and some of civilian cases, give an idea of how they may arise.

Driver J., while on duty in France, was thrown from a horse and struck his head. He was unconscious for a time and was told that he had a fit. He recovered quickly, but after coming round he had a severe headache. Six months later, while grooming his horses, he again had a severe headache. He was much fatigued and under considerable emotional strain at the time, and the headache was followed by a fit. Subsequently he had frequent fits, but these only occurred when he had a severe headache. In this case the sensational pattern of headache had become associated with the motor pattern of a fit, and whenever he had a severe headache a fit was suggested and took place.

M., a microcephalic of low intelligence, was a very " frightened " boy and an obvious misfit in life. Whenever anyone came at all noisily into the room he was in, he had a fit. This proved to depend upon a memory dating from childhood, and when he was made to realize this, his fits ceased at any rate for the time. He had had a drunken father who used to cause him great alarm when he came into the house and knocked things about. On these occasions he would run to his mother's arms, where he would have a convulsion, which apparently was an overflow of muscular activation due to the inhibition of complete flight. This is analogous to the case described above in relation to tics, in which, however, the emotional disposition was sex and not fear, as in the present case.

A similar case is the following : Sergt. W. was a machine-gunner and had his post in the upper story of a ruined house. One day a shell scored a direct hit on the house, and when he came to himself W. found that he had fallen through the floor to the ground. When he picked himself up he could not speak. He went outside, where he met a medical officer and endeavoured to describe the occurrence to him, but, being unable to speak, could tell him nothing. In the course of his attempts he became extremely agitated, until finally he fell down in a fit. Again activity, inhibited in one direction, finds outlet in some other direction, and in this case did so in the purposeless movements of a fit. This patient subsequently developed temporary aphonia on frequent occasions. This was followed by twitching of one side of his face, and on two occasions which were observed, the activity spread till a complete convulsion occurred. Investigation showed that the aphonia was preceded by a thought or mental image of the war and of his primary accident, and, although in this case a complete fit was not always produced, it is easy to see how such a suggestion would perpetuate a series of hysterical convulsions.

Hysterical fits may result from imitation. Thus Hurst quotes a case of a soldier servant, who had seen his officer killed, the latter dying after some convulsive movements. The servant thereupon had a fit, and this was repeated on subsequent occasions. The nature of hysterical fits will be determined by what the patient thinks a fit ought to be like. The man who knows nothing about epilepsy will simply throw himself down and wave his limbs about in a more or less violent manner. As is the case with so many hysterical symptoms, this action will be as obvious and theatrical as possible, so that the movements may become extremely violent and require considerable force to restrain them. Although the action is not within the control of the active consciousness, it is guided by a certain degree of integration of emotional dispositions, so that self-preservation prevents injury to the person, with the result that the patient always has his fit on the grass or on a bed where he is unlikely to hurt himself. I once saw a large crowd of neurotic patients assembled on a gravel square surrounded by grass plots. A statement was read out, which caused them considerable emotional excitement. About five or six had fits, and not one of these fell on to the gravel ; without exception they managed to reach the grass before they collapsed.

In patients who are familiar with what a true epileptic fit really is, by reason of having suffered from them in their own persons or having closely observed others afflicted with this disease, the diagnosis may be much more difficult. Here the movements may exactly simulate true epilepsy, and the well-known diagnostic signs of this condition, such as tongue-biting and involuntary micturition, cease to hold good. Such men know that the tongue is bitten in epilepsy, and they will unconsciously bite their tongues and lips sufficiently to cause bleeding, but the injury is never extensive, and the deep scars, sometimes observed in true epileptics, are not seen in hysterical cases. Similarly, these patients know that epileptics pass their urine while in a convulsion, and this they will do during the hysterical fit. Rarely, epileptics relax their anal sphincter ; this never happens in hysterical cases.

The cases referred to as having had epilepsy themselves, will include two groups. Firstly, those who have had true epilepsy in childhood or early adult life, but in whom the disease has apparently ceased, until the occurrence of an emotional crisis, when the fits reappear. These latter fits will in many cases prove to be hysterical and therefore curable. Secondly, one cannot study a series of cases of true epilepsy, without being struck by the frequency with which the condition is complicated by the occurrence of hysterical fits. Presuming that it is right to say that an hysterical fit is caused by suggestion, what can be more suggestive than a true epileptic fit ? This will be the case especially if the fit is accompanied by an aura. For example, if the aura consists in a tingling of the fingers, whenever the fingers tingle, from whatever cause, a fit will be suggested, and, if the patient is susceptible, he will have one.

The following cases exemplify these conditions :

A. R. had fits when a baby, which continued until he was eight years old and then ceased. At the age of twenty-one, when in Egypt, the fits returned and persisted for eighteen months. He had no more until called for Army service at the age of forty-two. He was then much disturbed over business matters, and found the training very hard. He developed fits, which were cured by psychotherapy. In this case the fits during childhood were almost certainly due to true epilepsy ; the nature of those at the age of twenty-one is doubtful, but those at the age of forty-two were clearly hysterical.

Pte. J. had had fits all his life, some of which were clearly true epilepsy, and one observed was definitely so. After a bad time in France, his fits became much more frequent and he had two or three a week. The majority of these were manifestly hysterical, and as a result of psychotherapy a period of two months passed without a fit. This was a longer interval free from convulsions than he had enjoyed in civil life.

Pte. H. was wounded by a shell on August 1, 1918, in the back, thigh and scalp. There was no fracture of the skull, and all wounds had healed five weeks later, and ten weeks after the wound no scar could be found in the scalp. It was clear, however, that he had been concussed at the time of the wound and had had a short period of unconsciousness. Since the wound, he had had a series of fits at intervals varying from two days to two weeks. He professed complete ignorance of these fits, and stated that he had been brought in on more than one occasion by some passer-by, who had discovered him lying unconscious on the road, and that he knew nothing as to how the fit began or what happened except what was told him. Such a history points to the fits being organic in nature. However, he did not relax his sphincter or bite his tongue, and had no aura, while on one occasion he was apparently very violent, six men being required to hold him down. These facts point rather to an hysterical fit, and it is probable that his was one of the mixed cases described above. He was treated by psychotherapy and at the same time given bromide ; he was discharged from hospital, having been seven weeks without a fit, more than three times the length of his previous record.

When hysterical fits closely simulate true epilepsy there are only two signs which will certainly establish a diagnosis. The most important of these is the presence of an extensor plantar reflex after the termination of the fit. If this is definitely found, the fit is one of true epilepsy, but unfortunately this sign is not always present in organic fits, and at best its presence is fleeting, disappearing almost immediately after the return of consciousness. To be of diagnostic value the sign must be quite definite. Secondly, Collier and Buzzard lay stress on conjugate deviation of the eyes in organic epilepsy ; this is said not to occur in hysterical fits. For the rest we must be guided by other signs, which although not pathognomonic, yet taken together will form valuable corroborative evidence in influencing our decision. The history of the onset is often valuable, definite association with emotional crises or strong suggestive influences being in favour of hysteria. The frequency of the fits and the conditions under which they occur are important. Very great frequency suggests that some at least of the fits are hysterical. Occurrence in connexion with emotional crises or with some particular symptom, with which they were associated in the first instance, is in favour of hysteria. It has been stated that fits occurring at night are not likely to be hysterical, but this is by no means always true, as I have seen cases where hysterical fits occurred at night, the emotional origin being afforded by a dream. Moreover, many so-called fits are really somnambulisms. In true epilepsy the patient is not violent and does not require to be held down by force, but often in hysterical fits the movements are very violent and the patient will relate that several men were required to restrain him. In spite of all this apparent violence the patient seldom hurts himself, and the hysteric does not present the scars and bruises of the true epileptic.

Post-epileptic automatism does not occur after hysterical fits, but it is not at all impossible for an hysterical fit to occur in conjunction with a fugue, which might be practically indistinguishable from post-epileptic automatism, so that it is impossible to lay down any hard and fast rule on this point.

It is necessary to point out that fits may be consciously feigned. They will vary with the subject's conception of what epilepsy ought to be like, just as is the case in the hysteric, but the malingerer has to put himself to a much greater strain to maintain his rôle, and consequently if under close observation he may be forced to confess his deceit, and the tramp with the soap in his mouth does not deceive the trained observer.

Hysterical Gaits.—These are of all varieties ranging from methods of progression, whose very grotesqueness stamps them as obviously hysterical to close imitations of the well-known gaits of organic disease. The former variety usually depends on various local rigidities or paralyses of muscle groups, which will throw the limbs into curiously abnormal relationships. For example, in a case of slight genu valgum, a synovitis of the affected knee was followed by rigidities and relaxations of the surrounding muscles, which so far exaggerated the habitual knock-knee that his legs, when he walked, assumed the shape of a capital K. However, a very short course of re-education and persuasion sufficed to restore him to normal.

The dancing gait of the spastic hysteric is common and quite characteristic, but it has often been observed that after repeated examinations by different physicians, the gait, as well as the whole appearance of the patient, comes to simulate closely that of an organic spastic paraplegia. Similarly, the ataxia of tabes may be very closely mimicked, either as the result of imitation of a genuine case, or as the result of the hetero-suggestion of the examining physician. In such cases, we usually find Rombergism is present, and often certain anæsthesias, but there are of course no reflex changes, no Argyll-Robertson pupil and no change in the vibration sense.

Another gait commonly produced by hetero-suggestion is that of the tilted pelvis. A spasm of the pelvic muscles has produced limping in the corresponding limb. Measurements of the limb have been carelessly taken, and the man told that he has shortening and a special boot ordered. This of course perpetuates the spasm and the abnormal gait continues. Further, the very spasm of the muscles produces pain. Pain may produce further tilting, and so the symptom is indefinitely perpetuated. Once the true nature of these conditions is discovered, treatment is, as a rule, a simple matter. A perpetuation of the spasm of the ilio-psoas, which occurs in appendicular and pelvic inflammatory states, is not uncommon, and is sometimes responsible for the persistent pain and limps which occur after abdominal operations. These are all further illustrations of the same principles as have been referred to above.

Hysterical Disorders of Speech.—The three most common functional disorders of speech are mutism, aphonia and stammering, though rarely others do occur. Aphasia is very rare, but may be simulated in cases of extreme regression when the mode of speech of the infantile period is released. A case of a sergeant was met with, whose whole behaviour had regressed to a very low level and who during his waking movements could only make sounds which were like those of an aphasic ; while asleep, however, he was capable of calling out military orders in the most approved parade voice, much to the alarm of other patients sleeping near him. Déjérine [1] notices that " one sometimes meets a group of symptoms, which more or less resemble motor aphasia, but the power of writing is almost always completely retained. If agraphia

[1] Déjérine and Gauckler, *Les Manifestations Fonctionelles des Psychonévroses.* Paris 1911.

occurs, which is rare, it is total, and all forms of writing are affected. On the other hand a very small number of cases of sensory aphasia and pure word deafness have been noticed among hysterics." Ripman [1] has described a case of hysterical idioglossia in a soldier, a condition in which the patient seems to speak a distinct language of his own, substituting alternative sounds for the consonants, but producing the vowels correctly.

Mutism may or may not be associated with deafness, and in the vast majority of cases it follows an emotional shock.

Déjérine, before the war, described the pathogenesis of the condition, and experience has confirmed his observation : " Les malades sous l'influence de l'émotion ont perdu leur voix. Ils ne savent plus le retrouver parce que la conviction de leur impuissance les empêche de la rechercher."

Mutism occurs early in the history of a neurosis and is usually recovered from more or less completely in a short time. Amongst over three hundred neurotics under my personal care during the latter part of hostilities, very few of whom came direct from France, I did not have a single mute patient, though several stammerers and aphonics had been mute and developed these other symptoms in the course of a partial recovery.

When mutism occurs, it is complete and corresponds to no organic condition. The hysterical mute utters no sound whatever, either in laughing, whistling, or coughing, whereas the aphasic patient—the only condition with which mutism may be conceivably confused—can always articulate some sounds, though these may not be intelligible. Further the mute can express by means of gestures or writing perfectly lucid accounts of his experience, but this is not the case in aphasia. Hurst, however, notes a case of a mute who could not write, but expressed himself quite clearly by drawing. Mutes frequently call out in their dreams, and the frequency of their recovery

[1] C. Ripman, *Seale Hayne Neurological Studies.* Oxford 1918.

as the result of a new emotional shock, or when a chance word strikes an association highly charged with emotional tone, is too well known to require detailed description, but one example may be allowed. A patient who had been mute presented documents in which he was noted as cured as the result of treatment in a certain hospital. Investigation showed that the " treatment," which had cured his mutism, was a fall down sixty stone steps.

As has been stated, aphonia often occurs in patients who have been incompletely cured of mutism, but by far the commonest cause is laryngitis. This actually deprives the patient of the power of phonation for a period of a few days or a few weeks. The patient, finding he cannot phonate, accepts the suggestion that this is permanent, and remains aphonic for months or even years. The same condition may ensue as the result of ether anæsthesia or infective inflammation of the tonsils or larynx.

Stammering may originate in the course of recovery from mutism, or as a result of emotional shock, or by imitation. Roussy and Lhermitte [1] attempt to discriminate between real stammering and hysterical stuttering, but it would appear that all stammering is hysterical, whether it is acquired in early life or later on. As in all hysterical symptoms, we must recognize the suggested factor and the physical and mental phenomena which ensue. With regard to the former, we know that rigidity of the muscles is one of the essential expressions of the emotions of fear and anger. If then, as a result of a sudden emotional shock, the muscles of respiration and voice production become rigid, stammering will follow as a temporary secondary expression of the emotion, since the phenomenon of stuttering depends on the rigidity of these muscles. If the suggestion thus presented is accepted, as it may well be in the confused state of the patient's mind, the condition will become a fixed hysterical symptom.

[1] Roussy and Lhermitte, *The Psychoneuroses of War*. London 1918.

The physical manifestation of stammering will be found to consist in the rigidity and wrong use of the muscles of respiration of the larynx and of the mouth. As a rule all these groups of muscles are at fault together, but one or other may predominate. If the chest muscles are at fault, the patient fails to get anything out at all at first, and then the sentence comes with a rush, the words tumbling over each other in the attempt to get them out, before the breath stops again. If the laryngeal and palatal muscles are chiefly at fault, there will be difficulty over initial vowels, and there will be the harsh monotonous tone in the voice, which is so characteristic of stammerers, while, if the action of the labial muscles is spasmodic, stuttering over initial consonants will be the chief feature of the condition. The respiratory exchange of the stammerer is almost always deficient, and furthermore he does not use what breath he has correctly. In voice production phonation should occur during expiration, but the stammerer either tries to produce his voice during inspiration, or when there is no breath in the lungs, or when the breath is held.

Often in addition to the spasm of the muscles involved in speaking, there is a " tic " of all the facial muscles, so that the patient makes the most strange grimaces, when he tries to talk, and in severe cases the arms or even the whole body may share in the universal inco-ordination of muscular action. Almost more important than these physical symptoms of stammering is the mental factor, which consists in the development of the dread of stammering. The patient loses confidence in his ability to get his words out, and this makes him try to rush his words before breath fails him. This accounts for the fact that all stammerers speak too fast. This mental symptom is the one which is the most resistant to treatment, and many a stammerer feels a dread of not being able to get out certain words, but by means of some trick manages to avert disaster, and prevents his infirmity being discoverable to a casual acquaintance. One patient of mine who had a very slight stammer amongst other neurotic symptoms had a dread of certain words, but was often able to see these coming in the sentence he was speaking, and having a somewhat agile mind was able to substitute some other form of expression, and thus avert the disclosure of his disability.

Hysterical Pain.—This is a subject of great complexity, for it is obviously very difficult to estimate the severity of a pain which is entirely subjective. In dealing with hysterical pain, we may leave on one side the headache of fatigue subsequent to emotional excess. True hysterical pains are those which are directly or indirectly the result of suggestion. As examples of pains which are a direct result, we have cases of painful scars, persistent pains after abdominal operations, headaches persistent after concussion and neuralgias following bruises or inflammation of peripheral nerves. Frequently, such pains will disappear as the result of psychotherapeutic treatment, which detracts the attention of the patient from himself. Indeed, it is often the case that the only way to determine the diagnosis is by the application of this therapeutic test. As an example of the indirect results of suggestion, the pain accompanying the various hysterical contractures may be cited. In such we have to deal with muscles in a condition of spasm which are exerting abnormal tension on their attachments. This may result in considerable pain, which is at once relieved by teaching the patient to relax his muscles. This state of affairs frequently explains the persistence of pain round joints which have been the seat of inflammatory changes. The patient still complains of pain long after all inflammation has subsided, and the condition comes to be described as chronic rheumatism, or by some other equally vague term, and the patient is dismissed without further trouble being taken with him. Before dismissing anyone who complains of pain, but in whom careful investigation fails to elicit an adequate cause, we must consider his sensitivity to stimuli. This matter is discussed elsewhere, so need not be dwelt on here, but as a rule this is a symptom which requires attention and treatment. A pain which has become useful to the patient in avoidance of duties or acquisition of sympathy, sometimes persists as a habit which is very difficult to break.

Hysterical Disorders of Common Sensation.—The various anæsthesias and hyperæsthesias have received far more attention than they deserve, because of the stress laid upon them by Charcot and his immediate followers as stigmata of hysteria. The doctrine of stigmata still finds credence amongst a large number of physicians and the principal stigmata in the classical descriptions of hysteria were various anæsthesias, which could be discovered by examining an hysterical patient, whether he presented other symptoms or not. These anæsthesias were peculiar, inasmuch as they did not cause the patient any inconvenience, and were not realized by him till pointed out by the physician. In 1900, Babinski[1] first attacked this doctrine, and pointed out that the anæsthesias, like the other stigmata of hysteria, were not present until they had been suggested by the examining physician. At most, they proved the suggestibility of the patient. But since every individual is suggestible, and on some occasions more so than others, this discovery proves nothing.

Another group of hysterical anæsthesias is, however, more difficult to decide upon. These are the cases following organic anæsthesias which are perpetuated by auto - suggestion, although the determining cause no longer operates. The commonest of these is the sequel of damage to peripheral nerves. After the nerve has been restored to function the anæsthesia is found to persist in some cases, and even to be responsible for burns or other accidents. The only way in which such persistent anæsthesia can be positively proved

[1] J. Babinski, *Gaz. des Hôpit.*, LXXVIII, pp. 521 and 533. 1900.

to be hysterical is by the therapeutic test, and this has been done in several such cases. Such anæsthesias often constitute a real disability, as for example when they prevent a workman handling his tools. Therefore, when such a case is met with and the restoration of muscular movement and trophic tone points to complete recovery of nerve function, were it not for the persistence of anæsthesia, the test of treatment should be applied. The same auto-suggestive disturbances of sensation will occur after vascular disorders involving the occlusion of blood-supply to a part. This may be caused by wounds or other injuries, by too tight bandaging or by the lowering of temperature with consequent vaso-constriction complicated by immobility and disuse. This should be considered in the same way as are nerve injuries, and in any case the resultant disability will be negligible, unless it involves the extremities in such a way as to interfere with the proper use of tools.

Hyperæsthesias arise in exactly the same way as anæsthesias and must be considered on the same lines, so that repetition is needless. All that need be said, is to reaffirm the law that the less attention paid to any disorders of common sensation the better for all concerned.

Hysterical Disorders of Vision.—The disorders of sight are not very uncommon and vary in severity from complete blindness to slight asthenopia.

The classical visual stigmata of restricted or distorted fields of vision for coloured or white light, which figure so largely in the writings of Charcot and the earlier French observers, are undoubtedly the outcome of hetero-suggestion. There is no such contracted vision until it is produced by the examining physician, and personally I have seen this stigma produced by a medical officer in the course of his examination.

The organic restriction of the visual field results in considerable difficulty in orientation, but this is not experienced in hysterical cases, hence by observation of the patient's

o

behaviour, it is possible to make a diagnosis without resorting to such elaborate diagnostic methods as perimetrical examination, since this will only tend to fix the idea of disability in the mind of the hysteric.

Complete blindness results from two psychogenic sources : firstly, there are the cases whose occipital lobes have received temporary injury by concussion or other means. These have a period of real organic blindness, but as the effect of the injury completely or partially passes off, the blindness continues as the result of auto-suggestion. It is an obvious truism that in order to see we must look, and if the effort to look has not resulted in seeing things, the suggestion of blindness may be accepted. The patient ceases to look and consequently does not see even when he might. Secondly, there are cases, whose eyes have been irritated by some external agency, as, for instance, by chemicals or by dust particles. The result of this is conjunctivitis with protective closing of the eyes. This closing of the eyes may persist after all inflammation has passed off, and may be met with as a tonic or clonic blepharo-spasm or as paralytic ptosis. Under these circumstances the patient will complain of blindness.

It may be mentioned in passing that the old distinction between organic and functional ptosis has been proved to be without value. Most text-books state that the frontalis is thrown into spasm as a result of an attempt to open the eyes in organic ptosis, but that this does not occur in functional ptosis.

A case of mine had ptosis and unilateral blindness, and his forehead was most markedly corrugated, especially on the blind side. The history, the nature of the condition and the rapidity of cure conclusively showed that this was hysterical in nature. This type of hysterically blind person keeps his eyes shut, and if they are forcibly opened, the balls roll upwards under the lids, so that he really does not see. Treatment consists in teaching the patient to recontrol the intrinsic and extrinsic muscles of the eye and to look. In the majority of cases with or without blepharospasm or ptosis the condition is bilateral, but when it is unilateral there is always an actual or an imagined weakness of the eye involved. For example one case of unilateral blindness had had styes in the affected eye ever since childhood, another stated that the eye then blind had always tended to get red and to water.

Asthenopia, fatigue and weakness of the eye is a very frequent accompaniment of neurosis of all sorts. It is a true hysterical symptom, being produced by the auto-suggestion of the patient or by the hetero-suggestion of excessive use of dark glasses or eye-shades.

Hysterical diplopia is not uncommon; it generally occurs as a perpetuation of a temporary organic diplopia. For example, a patient received a blow on the orbit with apparent slight damage to the superior rectus muscle, producing diplopia on looking upwards. Sometime after the objective signs of the superior rectus paralysis had passed off, he retained the subjective diplopia which was proved (by the rapidity of cure) to be an hysterical perpetuation. Such conditions as micropsy, megalopsy and the like have been described, but are too rare to merit discussion, and in all respects correspond to those referred to above.

In cases of hysterical disorders of vision, ophthalmological examination is necessary to establish a diagnosis, but this should only be carried out a minimum number of times, for, if the condition is hysterical, repeated examination only fixes the idea of disability in the patient's mind.

Hysterical Disorders of Hearing.—Hyperaceusis, in the sense of markedly increased sensitiveness to sounds so as to be actually painful, is a common accompaniment of the general irritable condition of the nervous system of all neurotics, but cases in which the capability of detecting sounds is actually increased are rare. Hurst had a case during the war, who could hear whispered conversation through shut doors to a degree which was estimated to be sixteen times greater than the normal. How this was brought about unless it was a hitherto undiscovered freak, which the patient had unconsciously possessed all his life, is difficult to say, as attempts to increase the powers of hearing in individuals by training have not usually been more successful than would be explicable by the increased power of attention

All degrees of deafness are commonly met with, and all depend on the fact that in order to hear it is necessary to listen, and in hysterical deafness the patient does not listen, just as in hysterical blindness he does not look. Deafness is frequently associated with mutism and sometimes with blindness. In the former case the cure of the mutism often results in the cure of the deafness at the same time. Where this is not the case, or where deafness occurs alone, treatment by persuasion or suggestion will be found successful, and in this particular hysterical symptom the grossest forms of suggestion have been claimed to be remarkably successful. One has known cases where "fake" operations, such as skin incision over the mastoid under incomplete ether anæsthetic have succeeded where all other methods have failed, but such practice should only be undertaken as a last resort, for failure in this case is final and complete, since the patient cannot be got to believe that his trouble is curable when an operation has not been successful.

One of the most difficult problems that faces the neurologist is to distinguish between hysterical deafness and malingering on the one hand and hysterical and organic deafness on the other. So far as malingering is concerned, unless the patient has been detected, able to hear one moment and not the next, it is well to be frank and admit that we cannot distinguish between this hysterical symptom and malingering. Still, if observation shows marked variation which corresponds to the pleasure or discomfort evoked by the patient's occupation at the time, one may at least conclude that he is not trying his best to get well. In a case of partial deafness, if the degree of disability seems to be in excess of the manifest changes and to vary from time to time in accordance with attention which the patient is paying, the hysterical nature of the condition should be presumed, and treatment may be of use if the patient is willing to keep on listening, but the strain of this is great and many people find it simpler to accept defeat, stop listening, and let the world pass by in silence.

In case of total deafness, most text-books lay down definite differentia to distinguish between organic and hysterical deafness. Babinski, for example, states that hysterical symptoms do not exist in sleep, but while some hysterically deaf patients are awakened by loud noises, I have seen others who have peacefully slept through the veriest pandemonium, produced in one case by a thunder-storm and in another by a big drum. Oppenheimer and others lay stress on the blink reflex. A normal person when he hears a loud noise automatically blinks his eyes. In the case of complete organic deafness, this is always lost, while hysterics are said to retain it. The controlling centre of this reflex has been proved to be in the mid-brain and it is natural to accept the view that, as hysterical deafness is a dissociation of the cortical function of listening, this mid-brain reflex is retained. However, I have seen cases which have been proved to be hysterical by their subsequent rapid cure by psychotherapy, in whom the dissociation has evidently extended to deeper levels, for this blink reflex was completely absent before cure, however loud a noise was produced, and returned immediately the cure was effected. One test however, seems to be of use, though I have seen a case recently, which throws doubt on the validity of even this method of detection. I refer to the various varieties of labyrinthine tests which are normal in the hysterically deaf patient. The rotation tests are the most readily applied and require no special apparatus for the purpose of rapid diagnosis. The most useful is that in which the patient stooping down rests his head on his hand, which grasps the top of an ordinary walking-stick; he is then rotated five times in one direction, he is raised to the upright position and told to walk straight forward. In normal and hysterical cases he will stagger towards the side to which he was rotated. But in organic nerve deafness involving the labyrinth he walks straight ahead without difficulty. He should be tested by rotation in both directions, and any difference in degree of stability noted. If this test is positive, we may be pretty confident that the condition is organic and not hysterical.

Hysterical Disorders of the Digestive System.—1. Hysterical Anorhexia.—The refusal of food has long been a familiar symptom of hysteria. The condition ranges from an almost normal idiosyncrasy resulting in a repulsion for certain types of food, to a complete refusal of all food of any sort. This latter condition is of really serious import and may even lead to death. The symptom is usually accompanied by vomiting of any food which is forced down, and the most profound wasting may eventually occur, though this is not so rapid as would be the case if the condition was organic. Vomiting and anorhexia of hysterical origin are very frequently diagnosed wrongly, and cases are labelled gastritis, although chemical or radiographic examination of the stomach shows no lesion which could account for the symptoms. Hurst maintained that all cases of the vomiting of pregnancy are hysterical and that they can all be cured by suggestion and persuasion, if this is sufficiently vigorous and confident. Whether we can go all the way with him in this may be open to doubt, but there is no question that he is right in many cases. Persistent vomiting after anæsthetics has also proved to be hysterical in some cases by the test of the successful psychotherapeutic treatment. In this type of case the presence of vomiting sug-

gests its continuance, and this is only stopped when the suggestion is countered.

Acute abdominal conditions, such as appendicitis, may often
suggest vomiting, which persists almost indefinitely, and the
following case is typical of such.

H. B. developed acute appendicitis and was operated on
and the appendix removed at once. Vomiting and right iliac
pain persisted however, and six weeks later his abdomen was
again opened for supposed adhesions. After this, vomiting
became worse rather than better, and shortly before his admission to hospital, he had been fed by nutrient enemata, all food
by the mouth being withheld, and opium was actually being
given for the pain. Three days' persuasive treatment sufficed
to restore him to full diet and to relieve the pain completely.
Although he had two relapses which were of great interest in
view of their cause, since the symptom was revived as a temporary way out of an unpleasant emotional situation in both
cases, he subsequently completely recovered, and six months
later he wrote that he was in perfect health, working full time
as a solicitor's clerk and going to dances most nights.

In this case it is clear that the persistence of symptoms was
the result of suggestion, and the same is probably true of many
cases of persistent vomiting, after various acute conditions in the
abdomen. It is to be noticed, too, that where reflex vomiting
occurs in such maladies as phthisis or chronic appendicitis,
the amount of vomiting may be very sensibly diminished
by psychotherapy, thus proving that some of the trouble is
hysterical. While this does not, of course, preclude the
treatment of the underlying condition, nevertheless it is
important that this should be kept in mind, both from the
point of view of the patient's comfort and of the prognostic
significance of his symptoms.

Emotions, and especially the emotion of disgust, is frequently the source of the suggestion. After the war it was by

no means rare to meet men who had vomited off and on ever since they were engaged on some repulsive task such as burying decomposed bodies, or since they encountered some repulsive sight, such as a corpse disembowelled by an explosive shell.

Gastric flatulence is very frequently of hysterical origin. The patient, for some reason or other, feels fullness in his stomach and this may have induced the natural expulsion of air swallowed with the food, which normally comes after a meal. He concludes that his feelings were due to flatulence and makes the effort to expel more gas. In so doing, he swallows more air than he brings up and so the process may go on indefinitely. Robert Hutchison particularly has drawn attention to this air-sucking. Hiccup is another hysterical manifestation that is met with from time to time, and psychotherapy is sometimes useful even in the exhausting hiccup of intestinal obstruction, if the patient is not too ill to respond.

The last hysterical condition of the digestive system which merits description is a form of constipation which is very common in all ranks of society and in both sexes. This is what Hurst [1] has described as " dyschezia." In such cases, radiographic investigation shows that the waste material of digestion reaches the pelvic colon in the normal time, but that it is held up here. Normally, fæces accumulate in the pelvic colon, the rectum remaining empty until a certain pressure is reached. When this occurs, the pelvi-rectal flexure is passed, there is a call to stool in normal individuals, not on account of irritation of the mucous membrane, which is insensitive, but of the stimulation of the muscle sense, induced by dilation of the tube. Hurst's experiments showed that the call to stool occurred when the pressure in the viscus reached a certain constant figure ; but if this was neglected, the pressure fell, owing to the relaxation of the muscles. It

---

[1] A. F. Hurst, *Constipation and Allied Intestinal Disorders*, p. 142. London 1919.

therefore required a further accumulation of fæces to restore the pressure requisite to induce the call to stool. If this was again neglected, the process went on till almost complete atony of the rectum resulted with consequent severe constipation. Conditions of modern life are such that the call to stool is frequently neglected, with the result that dyschezia is produced. As the patient begins to feel the local and general discomfort of accumulating fæcal material, he has recourse to salts or the omnipresent purgative pill which can always be obtained from the nearest chemist's shop. The action of these purgatives is to hurry fæcal material from the small intestine through the colon and this carries away the hard fæces with it on evacuation. This induces the suggestion of severe constipation, which can only be relieved by purgatives, and a vicious circle is set up, for the more the purgatives are taken the firmer becomes the suggestion, and the firmer the suggestion, the more apparent need for purgation. Persuasive and re-educative treatment readily relieves the trouble by reinstituting proper habits and substituting lubricants and rectal stimulants for purgatives. In many cases the health of the individual is very materially benefited, for the too rapid action of the bowels prevents the proper absorption of the food and failure of nutrition ensues.

Hysterical Disorders of the Cardiac and Respiratory Systems.—The neuropathic disturbance of these systems is probably most accurately described as prolonged expression of emotion, such as is the disordered action of the heart so common in the war, for it is doubtful if a symptom should be regarded as hysteria unless it is one which conceivably can be imitated consciously. At the same time, emotional expression often forms the basis of a suggestion and the symptom is continued as an hysterical manifestation. Disturbances of both systems are frequently met with accompanying other hysterical symptoms, such as fits and gross tremors, but isolated cardiac disturbances can hardly be regarded as truly hysterical. However, so far as the respiratory system is concerned, tachipnœa, coughing, and all sorts of groaning and barking respiratory noises are met with at times. There is generally not the slightest difficulty in recognizing these as hysterical and they should, of course, be dealt with as such.

Hysterical Disorders of the Reproductive System.—The various forms of sexual impotence are relatively common hysterical symptoms, and may or may not be accompanied by spermatorrhœa, which is probably a secondary result of emotional disturbance. These symptoms are always accompanied by marked manifestations of anxiety which may be the cause or the result of the impotence. So great a mental influence do these symptoms have that serious depression is not an infrequent result. Although the symptom itself cannot perhaps be regarded as responsible for preventing a man from earning his living, the mental effects certainly do disable him, and treatment is difficult, since the methods of cure by persuasion and re-education are not applicable as in other hysterical conditions. The treatment must deal with the anxiety elements of the case, and the prognosis depends on the severity of these.

As to the origin of this group of symptoms, the suggestion may be started by an actual failure in the performance of the sexual act as the result of fatigue, local pain or other cause. In other cases an operation such as circumcision, excision of a hydrocele or varicocele will sometimes induce a suggestion of damage to sexual powers.

Fear of venereal disease in the man's own person or disgust and anger at discovering it in his wife may lead to the same result, but by far the commonest cause is the dread of the results of masturbation as portrayed by quack literature and even in would-be moral homilies. If punishment should fit the crime, then, in view of the mental torture they inflict on their victims, there is no depth of the inferno sufficiently terrible to house the authors of these publications.

Hysterical Disorders of the Urinary System.—The hysterical manifestations met with in connexion with this system are retention, abnormal frequency, precipitate micturition and incontinence of urine, both diurnal and nocturnal.

With regard to the two former conditions, most authorities are agreed that they are frequently hysterical, but incontinence has generally been regarded as organic. Moore,[1] however, has pointed out that many of these cases are hysterical, and a few patients suffering from this condition in my own experience have confirmed this, for treatment by psychotherapy has sufficed to cure them. How far incontinence continuing from infancy into later childhood is hysterical is a point which still requires clearing up, but it would seem that at least some cases, who are not mentally deficient, are of this nature and therefore, a trial of psychotherapeutic treatment is indicated. The genesis of the condition is frequently traumatic, injury to the bladder or urethra fixing the suggestion, after the actual trauma is recovered from. In other cases fear of getting disease and injudicious examinations by medical men are responsible for implanting the idea in the patient's mind. Lastly, persistence of emotional expression may determine the symptom. In all cases of disturbance of micturition, hysteria must be kept in mind when the organic lesion is inadequate to explain the condition. Certain cases of nocturnal enuresis have been shown to be due to a symbolic substitute for sexual gratification. This is rendered possible when higher levels of control are in abeyance during emotional conflict, when we consider how closely the vegetative nervous supply of the urinary and genital systems are associated in the pelvic

[1] J. W. Moore, *Hysterical Disorders of Micturition* (*Seale Hayne Neurological Studies*). Oxford 1918.

plexus, so that conditioning and redistribution of the pattern of activation is easily effected.

Hysterical Disorders of Memory.—Several varieties of memory defect are met with amongst neurotics, and the question as to which of them are hysterical is a difficult one. The commonest is the intermittent lapse of memory of the anxiety case, which is really a failure to recall, rather than an amnesia.

More difficult to discriminate are the amnesias associated with somnambulisms, fugues, and the like, in which certain phases of the patient's existence are forgotten during his " normal state."

These may resemble the hysterical amnesias closely, but are really symptoms of dissociation, and do not fit into the definition of hysteria here adopted, that symptoms are the product of suggestion. Again, there are the anterograde amnesias,—the loss of memory for recent events,—which are usually associated with certain psychoses, senility and, more usually, with the Korsikoff's syndrome of alcoholic poisoning. In the same class are the paramnesias, such as the phenomenon of *déjà vu*, which are due to false associations and unusual affective relationships with patterns of visual imagery.

What would seem to concern us here are the various retrograde amnesias which may be more or less complete. By this is meant a complete loss of memory for a certain period of life, which may be long or short. Very rarely, cases occur in which this is absolutely total, that is to say the subjects have not only lost the memory of who they are, where they live, etc., but also have completely lost all they ever knew and have to learn all their accomplishments *de novo*, how to read, to write, and even to walk and talk.

A much more common condition is a complete intellectual amnesia with retention of habitual requirements. These are the cases which sometimes come into the hands of the police, quite unable to account for themselves, having no recollection of their name, address, occupation, or events of their past life.

This leads up to the consideration of short periods of amnesia of a few hours to those of a few months' duration. Considerable controversy has taken place as to whether it is advisable or not to restore such amnesias. Personally, I think this restoration is essential in the treatment of the anxiety symptoms which accompany the loss of memory, for undoubtedly this type of amnesia is purposive in the Freudian sense, that is to say there is some event or situation, which the patient finds it is intolerable to remember. Theoretically such amnesia may occur, without anxiety symptoms, in which case, of course, it is advisable to leave well alone, but this desirable state of affairs is hardly ever met with, and in order to cure the anxiety the lost memories must be restored.

With reference to the cause of hysterical amnesia, it is often difficult to determine the exact psychic process which is responsible. Many cases however seem to correspond with hysterical blindness and deafness. A man is concussed and wakes up in a confused mental condition, or he may suffer from mental confusion of other kinds. He tries to remember and finds he cannot, and therefore accepts the idea that he has no memory and makes no further attempt to recall his experiences. This is similar to the way in which certain cases of blindness and deafness develop in patients, who try to see and fail, and therefore cease to look, or who try to hear and cannot and therefore cease to listen. The same sequence may result from the confusional state of mind, which occurs in acute emotional conflict or when repression has taken place, and the patient only succeeds with difficulty in preventing the entrance of the undesired pattern into the field of consciousness.

Hysterical Insomnia.—Insomnia in neurotics is a **very**

common symptom, but it is relatively rare that this is a true hysterical manifestation. In the vast majority of cases it is due to anxiety, and whenever dreams are present the insomnia must be considered as a symptom of this latter neurosis. The only cases, which can be classed as hysterical, are those in which there is no emotional disturbance, and there is a definite history of some suggestion which has operated as a cause and the insomnia has continued as a habit. In such cases hypnosis or the wise exhibition of hypnotics will cure the condition.

CHAPTER X

THE DISSOCIATION SYNDROMES

THE dissociation syndromes comprise the clinical conditions which were described by Janet [1] in his American lectures on the major symptoms of hysteria, namely the somnambulisms, fugues, and double personalities. In these the personality of the patient seems to change from time to time to a greater or less degree. What really happens is that the pattern which dominates the rest for the time being changes, and this pattern is sufficiently comprehensive·to achieve consciousness either to the exclusion of or coincidently with the rest of the personality. Such changes of dominating pattern are met with in ordinary life. McDougall [2] has shown that in the well-regulated individual the self-regarding sentiment is the dominating and controlling influence. Sentiments, however, may or may not be permanent, and may wax and wane according to the changed circumstances of the environment. Love and hate may be taken as good examples of sentiments, and, as Freud has shown, in the neurotic at any rate, there may be great instability in the dominance of either one or other even in respect of the same individual. This is specially the case in relation to childish emotional adjustments to parents or parent substitutes, love giving place to hate and hate to love without any very serious reason for the change. Similarly, in the love attachments, affection is given first to one individual

[1] P. Janet, *The Major Symptoms of Hysteria.* New York 1907.
[2] W. McDougall, *Social Psychology*. London 1917.

and then to another, so that the new love is approached, almost before the old one is dropped.

The simplest dissociation syndrome is the somnambulism. The patient who is subject to this may go on for considerable periods as an apparently normal individual, when suddenly his behaviour will change and he will perform certain acts and express certain emotions for a time and then equally suddenly will revert to his normal state again. On close examination, it is generally found that the somnambulism represents a pantomimic revival of an experience, which is entirely repressed and forgotten during the normal state. This corresponds to the state of affairs which is met with in some dreams, which represent, more or less symbolically, phantasies, attitudes and conations of which the patient is quite unaware in his waking state. The word "somnambulism" in its ordinary connotation implies a walking or other active behaviour during sleep, and this is probably merely a pantomimic representation of a dream. In the technical sense the term "somnambulism" is extended to similar pantomimic representations during the waking state, but there is no real essential difference between the two. The classical example is Janet's case of Irene, who, after her mother's death, seemed perfectly callous and forgetful of the event during her ordinary condition, but from time to time passed into another state, in which she showed expressions of uncontrollable grief. A similar case from my own experience is that of a man who on returning from the war developed "attacks," during which he lost all touch with his surroundings. If they occurred during the daytime, he would be unaware what he was doing or where he was going. Yet all the time he would walk along without stumbling. In other words, his habitual automatic actions were performed adequately, but his attention was directed elsewhere. During the attack he experienced fear and anxiety, and "expressed" these feelings in his general appearance. At the same time, he performed various gestures which were inexplicable, both to himself and to his companions. Later, it was possible to discover that during these " attacks " he was paying attention to a series of images, which were accompanied by emotional experience, and that the gestures he performed were appropriate to them. These images represented himself and his mother serving a company in a menial capacity. The host and hostess of this company were a banker and his daughter. To this daughter he had at one time been much attached, but monetary losses had resulted in a change in his social sphere which had made marriage impossible. As a rule, this set of ideas was seldom, if ever, in his mind, since he had done his best to repress it and dissociate it. That is to say, the group of emotional dispositions organized round his conception of himself in relation to his environment did not usually include this other subsidiary sentiment of love for the banker's daughter. But with a change in the orientation of the self-regarding sentiment, this love sentiment became dominant, to the exclusion of every other subsidiary sentiment. To put the state of affairs in another way, as a rule the general organization of his mental activities was towards his present recovery from the effects of the war, and his future means of livelihood. Suddenly, he would regress to a former state, in which the organization of his mental activities was towards marriage with the banker's daughter. Yet this regression was not complete, for in the phantasy he and his mother appeared in a menial capacity and not as equals with the banker and his daughter, and the fulfilment of his wish still seemed impossible.

It is to be noticed that these alternating patterns are mutually exclusive and that it is the purpose of treatment to bring them on to the level of reflective consciousness, at which the barriers between the patterns may be broken down and the whole integrated so as to eliminate conflict or dissociation within the personality. This may be done by the usual

P

methods of discovering the basis of the secondary states. Clues to this may be obtained from a close observation of the behaviour of the patient during such states, and sometimes from a study of a series of his dreams. In many cases however, hypnosis is a very useful means for discovering what is required, for under the influence of suggestion the secondary pattern may be so stimulated as to become dominant and achieve consciousness, so that the patient may be able to relate under hypnosis the whole story which determines the pattern. As a general rule, when the two patterns can be brought together, there is no difficulty in integration and the somnambulistic state associates itself with the rest of the personality. Until such cure is brought about the secondary pattern is apt to repeat itself indefinitely in these simple mono-ideistic somnambulisms. The different attacks are always exactly alike, repeating the same movements, expression and words over and over again and exerting no influence on ordinary consciousness. The change from one pattern to another is generally sudden and may be accompanied by severe pain in the head. What physical change this corresponds to is not certain, but there must be a profound modification of the synaptial junctions to induce sudden inhibitions of large patterns. Such biochemical changes may well be accompanied by vascular or other modifications such as might induce severe pain.

Mild degrees of somnambulisms are comparatively common and are often overlooked. Children are especially liable to this form of neurotic symptom. When it occurs in sleep, it is of course obvious, and is generally put down to indigestion or some other physical cause, but what is really happening is that the patient is experiencing a dream, the pattern of which is so comprehensive that motor tracts are involved and movements are carried out, which will be more or less organized and complex, according to the construction of the pattern. These movements are pantomimic representations of the emotional complex which is at the moment dominant. No better example could be afforded of this than the sleep-walking of Lady Macbeth. Somnambulisms occurring in children during the waking state are also common, but are not so readily recognized. In such conditions, the child may be apparently in a normal state, since he will respond to direct stimuli such as definite orders given expressly to him, and his incomprehensible behaviour in the intervals of performing these orders is put down to naughtiness or temper. For example, a girl of thirteen was told by a governess with whom she was on quite friendly terms to get out of bed in the morning. This she did, but she subsequently became rigid, seemed to be unaware of her surroundings, and when the governess took hold of her, the child struck out and hit her in the face. The latter then shook her and told her to go and wash herself. The child seemed to come to herself, said: " Where am I ? " and then quite naturally went to the bathroom. Close and intelligent observation demonstrated that she really was unaware of what had happened during the few moments of her " attack." Subsequent investigation showed that some time previously she had been intensely afraid of another teacher, and although she had never actually struck her, had been forming phantasies of doing so. On this occasion, as on others when similar behaviour took place, the firm command had been sufficient to activate the phantasy pattern, which had for the moment become dominant. It is not always recognized how easily such phantasy patterns may become dominant in children, especially if they are of the instable type. Moreover, the child is never so sure as to what is real and what is phantasy, as is the adult, and the pattern which is dominant for the moment does not so definitely exclude the rest of the personality as is the case in adult somnambulisms. Consequently a direct stimulus is able to reactivate other patterns, and temporarily or more permanently depose the phantasy pattern.

Similar " attacks " occur in adults and are often diagnosed as epileptic attacks or attributed to some other physical condition. Two examples will illustrate this. A man was subject to so-called epileptic attacks occurring when half asleep at night. During these he seemed to be utterly unconscious as far as external things were concerned, but had sufficient control of his motor functions to be able to get out of bed to pass water if occasion demanded during his apparent unconsciousness. He never hurt himself, bit his tongue or became incontinent, as happens in a genuine epileptic attack. His limbs did not move, but when he came to himself he felt dejected, his head was heavy and he felt good for nothing. Clearly these attacks were not epileptic, and investigation showed that they were really of the nature of a somnambulism, that they depended upon a very strong feeling of inferiority in which he blamed himself for various occurrences in childhood, chiefly concerned with masturbation. In this case, the association which activated the pattern responsible for the " attacks " was an emotional one of remorse and self-depreciation.

Another case was that of Capt. H., who complained of " attacks," which came on when his attention was not engaged in anything very definite. These attacks were the most prominent symptoms of his neurosis, and consisted of a feeling of intense cold with shivering, which was associated with considerable tremor. This was followed by a feeling of intense heat. The attacks lasted for a few moments, and most of the doctors he had consulted had made a confident diagnosis of malaria, when they heard the attacks described, especially as he had served in the Near East. However, when they came to investigate further, there was no history of malarial infection and no rise of temperature associated with the actual attacks. Careful investigation showed that they were specially liable to occur in association with despair of the future. This was rather a feature of his condition at the time, as he no longer felt that the career he had proposed before the war was a suitable one, and he saw no prospect of any other in his state of health and at his age. Meanwhile, he had the responsibility of a family, with all too few resources to support it. Seeking for an emotional association—that is to say, an event in which a similar emotion had been particularly intense—the real nature of the attack was explained. He had been severely wounded at Gallipoli and left for dead in front of a trench. A bullet had entered his neck and paralysed him in all his limbs from spinal concussion. He lay out for some hours fully expecting to die, and not extremely disturbed at the prospect in his semi-conscious state. Later, however, his lips were observed to move, and he was brought in. He was carried down to the beach in the evening and left there to be removed to a hospital ship. He was not taken off, however, for another twenty-four hours, so he lay exposed on a stretcher through a very cold night and an intensely hot day. During that time he was fully conscious, and the despair at being, as he felt, rescued from certain death in No Man's Land, only to be brought down and left to die on the beach, utterly overcame him. According to my explanation, during his attack, which was brought about by an emotional association, he re-enacted his sensations of extreme cold followed by intense heat endured during twenty-four hours in which the emotion of despair dominated his consciousness. Such a condition cannot, to my mind, adequately be explained by suggestion, and I prefer to regard it as a true somnambulism. It may be of interest to note, though admittedly this is of no value as to the accuracy of the theory, that on this explanation of his symptoms being given to the patient, he became a changed man. He again took an interest in life, slept well, could take exercise without fatigue, and generally became his old self. He chose a career which suited his tastes and took active measures to get himself trained for it.

The activation of the repressed pattern in these states is due to some association and the recognition of this is essential in treatment. In my rather limited experience the association is more often an emotional one than an ideational one.[1] By ideational association, I mean that the common factor which induces the attack is either an idea of the image of an object, while an emotional association is a feeling of some emotional state such as fear, anger, remorse, or the like. As a rule a careful examination of the mental activity preceding a series of such attacks in any patient will reveal some common factor which serves as the association, and this is the first necessity in treatment, in order that the whole process of conflict and dissociation in the patient's mind may be laid bare.

Fugues or Polyideistic Somnambulisms, as Janet has called them, do not differ from the simple somnambulisms, except in the complexity and comprehensiveness of the pattern. The temporarily dominant pattern governs the conduct of the individual for days or months together and may lead to a wandering away, so that he finds himself far from his home, without any conception as to how he got there. Such cases are not very common, but figure from time to time in the newspapers. The story is generally that an individual has been brought in by the police, having completely lost his memory. As this chapter is being written, the papers are full of the disappearance of a lady novelist who has caused a great stir by completely disappearing in the south of England and reappearing several days later in a northern town, apparently quite oblivious of what has happened. If the press reports can be relied upon, this does seem a good example of a fugue.

A case from my own experience is that of a lady who became very depressed and convinced of her own inadequacy, both to manage her own household and to attend to her religious

---

[1] Cf. Mr. Fortune in *The Mind in Sleep*, has pointed out how often this association pertains in dreams.

duties. While she was in this mood, she suddenly lost touch
with her surroundings and started to walk away. She had
only a few pence in her pocket, and these she spent on some
buns in a baker's shop. Finally she " came to herself " in a
village ten miles from home, in a very fatigued and foot-sore
condition. She had no knowledge of how she got there, nor
what she had done in the interval, and it was only afterwards
that the story of her walk and of the purchase of the buns was
elicited. Fugues of greater or less complexity were by no means
uncommon during the war, and in my own experience certain
cases of supposed desertion were recognized as such, just in
time before the extreme penalty was inflicted upon the patient.
In such circumstances the responsibility of medical officers
involved is an extremely grave one, for it is manifestly unjust
to punish a man for behaviour of which he is perfectly unconscious, but at the same time any general recognition of the
likelihood of such conditions being fugues would lead to widespread imitation. This is seen even in civil life, when a notorious
case of fugue, causing a great stir in the public imagination,
is apt to be followed by minor or less impressive cases, the
genuine nature of which is exceedingly hard to determine.
Again, it is necessary to point out that neurotics and children
are much less able than are normal adults to differentiate
between the various patterns, which from time to time occupy
consciousness, and are much more likely to behave in accordance with one or other to the exclusion of the rest of their
personalities. This is merely another way of saying that
their personalities are much less closely integrated and therefore dissociation is easy and frequent. The more neurones
involved in the production of any pattern of behaviour, the
less intense and violent will be that behaviour. It has already
been pointed out that the explanation of this lies in the resistance offered at the synaptial junctions to the spread of activation. It may be that, in these complicated alternations of

character, it would be better to express the change as one of orientation of the various affective and conative combinations within the self-regarding sentiment, rather than as the dominance of an entirely separate pattern, which would suppose the activation of a quite separate group of neurones. Hence the change might be more adequately expressed, by supposing the activation to flow over a different course amongst the neurones, and thus produce a new engram, though many of the actual neurones involved in the production of the rival patterns are the same.

This is specially so with the next group of cases, those of double personality. In these, the individual alternately presents two or more states, in which the personality differs profoundly. It sometimes happens that there is a complete amnesia for one state when the person is in the other; but often the condition is met with, to which Morton Prince has given the name co-consciousness.[1] In this there is complete awareness of the other state, through which the individual has passed.

I have not been fortunate enough to have had an actual case of double personality under my own observation, and as a matter of fact they are exceedingly rare. When they do occur they are of such great interest that they are fully reported, and most people are familiar with such cases as Dr Morton Prince's Sally Beauchamp [2] and the Rev. Anselm Bourne who, for most of his time, was a minister of religion in one town of the United States, but spent months on end carrying on a perfectly normal existence as a small grocer in another town. Since several of these cases are described very fully in psychological literature it is not necessary to go into them further here.

It is probable that the change of orientation within the sentiment is, at any rate partly, a product of endocrine

[1] Morton Prince, *The Unconscious.* Boston 1913.
[2] *Idem, The Dissociation of a Personality.* New York 1906.

activity, influencing the biochemical balance at the synaptial junctions. Such activities may be induced through the blood-stream, by what would be termed physical influences, such as fatigue products, poisons, etc., or may be induced by way of the central and sympathetic nervous systems, by what may be termed psychic influences, such as perceptions and images. The great difficulty in any such theory of action is of course to explain why an endocrine change, which presumably reaches all the synapses by way of the blood and cerebro-spinal fluid, should cause inhibition of one group and facilitation of another. Our answer can only be that we do not know. Yet it is quite clearly established in physiology that selective inhibition and facilitation do occur, as for instance in the simul-taneous contractions of the body, and relaxation of the neck of hollow viscera. Again, pharmacology teaches us that such drugs as curare, strychnine, etc., have a very specific action on certain very limited structures in the nervous system, and the analogy which we seek to draw does not seem impossibly far-fetched.

The treatment of these more complicated conditions is exactly the same as that of the simple somnambulisms, but is of course more difficult and takes much longer.

CHAPTER XI

EXHAUSTION NEUROSIS

FOR the sake of completeness, it is necessary to describe a condition to which the term " exhaustion neurosis " may be applied. This is the result of actual bodily or mental exhaustion. Cases were seen during the war after long and fatiguing retreats, and after extremely debilitating diseases. Many cases were seen after the retreat from Mons and some after the retreat in March 1918. Cases which occurred after the Russian retreat from the Donajecs and the Italian retreat from Capporetto have been described in continental literature. Exhaustion neurosis also occurred amongst men debilitated by diarrhœal diseases during the Gallipoli campaign. The result of these exhausting processes was to deprive the nerve cells of their proper nutrition, and on examination one would expect to find the individual cells shrunken and deficient in Nissl's granules.

So far as treatment was concerned, all that was necessary for these patients was that they should have rest and recuperation, and it was amongst such cases that this line of treatment, carried out by itself, was found to be completely effective.

The symptoms correspond in many ways to those of the milder cases of anxiety which depend on mental conflicts, but a diagnosis of exhaustion neurosis should only be made in the presence of a definite history of some exhausting factor which led to the condition, and a very short time should be sufficient to confirm or disprove the diagnosis thus made. In civil life, true uncomplicated exhaustion neurosis is rare, but in the case of business men, who have been grossly overworking, this may be the main causative factor, even though worries may be present as well, and the rest which restores the exhaustion factor is sufficient to enable them to cope with and overcome these worries. We must recognize, however, that fatigue is an important factor in the symptom formation of all varieties of neurosis. So long as the fatigue is due to friction between the ego as a whole and the outside world, the removal of the friction by isolation allows for the necessary recuperation, and recovery results. When, on the other hand, the fatigue is the result of friction within the ego, then mere rest is not enough, for the friction still persists, and cure does not ensue. It is a truism in neurology, that the higher structures are more readily fatigued than those of lower levels ; naturally therefore the functions of the cortical structures suffer first and most severely from any process of fatigue.

The conceptions of the functions of the cerebral cortex, the highest-grade structure in man, have changed not a little in recent years. With the tremendous impetus given to anatomical and histological study, by the improvements in optical and electrical methods, which took place in the last half of the nineteenth century, it seemed possible that the researches of such workers as Ferrier and Wernicke would lead to a mapping out of the whole cortex into geographical areas, each of which would be found to correspond to a definite function, connected with definite parts of the body. More recent work, however, has turned attention in other directions. Exact anatomical correspondence can no longer be regarded as part of the business of the cortex, though it is of course quite clear that certain areas have to do with certain major functions of the body, such as motion, sensation and the work of the distance receptors involving vision and hearing and so on. In these relations the functions to which cortical structure is essential are control, integration, discrimination and reference in time and space, as we have seen.

It has been remarked that the behaviour of neurotics, including those suffering from pure exhaustion neurosis, is mainly characterized by deficiency in what we have learnt to regard as the chief functions of the cortex. To take a few examples. In most hysterical paralyses, movements are impeded, not individual muscular action. It is characteristic of hysterical pain that the reaction, in some ways, resembles that seen in the thalamic syndrome, in which cortical control is absent. The behaviour of neurotics always tends to be of the " all-or-none " variety. This is especially true of their emotional reactions, which resemble to a certain extent those of Bianchi's monkeys,[1] whose frontal lobes were removed. Their undiscriminated anxieties and fears are primitive affective reactions, in no way co-ordinated into properly organized emotions and sentiments, and the resolution of these by the processes of psychotherapy essentially involves their proper discrimination and correlation. In the case of the obsessions, the salient feature is the want of accurate reference in time and space. So much is this so, that it is only by restoring the proper time-space relationship of these symptoms that they can be removed.

This may serve to indicate that the immediate precursor of neurotic symptoms is the abrogation of cortical function, and that this failure of function is to a certain extent due to the action of fatigue products. This conception does not run counter to other explanations of neurotic symptoms, such as conflict, repression, and dissociation, for the most marked forms of dissociation of function are those produced when the associative function of the cortex is in abeyance. Indeed, it is clear that a properly associated personality is only possible when the cortex is intact. It is, of course, the duty of the physician

---

[1] L. Bianchi, *Mechanism of the Brain and Function of the Frontal Lobes*. Edinburgh 1922.

not to be content with this explanation of symptoms, but to strive to discover the true cause of the fatigue ; by this means only will he cure the disease and not merely remove the symptom. None the less, the recognition that fatigue of the cortex is an important factor in this connexion is salutary, since it will tend to broaden the outlook of the physician, and prevent his applying only one method of treatment to all cases of neuroses. He will remember that fatigue may be induced by mental conflict, by a prolonged toxæmia, by endocrine disturbance, and by overwork, and so he is less likely to miss his view of the wood by too great concentration on individual trees. However, a very few weeks is ample for the recuperation of nerve cells, provided exhaustion is the only factor at work, that real rest can be obtained, and that no other process is interfering with recovery. Simple rest and good feeding should, therefore, be efficacious in a relatively short period of time if the diagnosis of exhaustion neurosis is a correct one. If by this time the symptoms have not cleared up, it is evident that some other factor is intervening, and it will be found, as a rule, that a mental conflict has got to be dealt with to ensure complete recovery.

In considering the symptoms of this condition, it must be remembered that such patients may readily acquire hysterical symptoms as the result of suggestion, but these have been dealt with under the general heading of Hysteria, and need not detain us here. The simple effects of exhaustion will be— a general subjective feeling of inefficiency and fatigue, a lack of power to concentrate or settle to any work, accompanied by headache, general malaise and sometimes a rather vague dizziness. Any other symptoms which may be present will be found to be of anxiety or hysterical origin, and will have to be dealt with by the more vigorous methods of analysis, suggestion or persuasion and re-education.

CHAPTER XII

THE PHYSICIAN AND THE PATIENT

I HAVE called this book The Neurotic Personality because I believe that the neurotic individual cannot be understood and cannot be helped unless his personality is appreciated. It may be remembered that the definition adopted here is that personality is an emergent, arising from all the bodily and mental structures and functions and all their relationships with the environment. It follows therefore, that if the physician is to understand and help the neurotic he must take a fairly comprehensive view of his patient.

Some people are apt to say that the neurotic would be much better without a physician, and that if he would discard all help and try harder to stand on his own feet he would get on better. This emphatically is not true. The neurotic is not guilty of want of effort, his efforts may be feeble, they are generally amazingly inadequate to meet the demands of life, but so far as in him lies, he is trying, although too often his efforts lead him in the wrong direction and are wasted. Frequently he is trying too hard and the first duty of the physician is to teach him to relax his efforts. He is like a young and frightened horse, dashing from side to side of a field trying to get out, although the gate is open, and the physician must go into the field, calm him down and lead him through the gate. This applies more obviously to the anxiety type than to the hysteric, for the latter often seems to regard his disability with considerable complacency, but this is only true if this hysterical symptom is adequately serving a definite purpose for the time being. Moreover, if we look a little deeper, we find he is not really satisfied—at least not for long—with the compromise which has been established. For example, during the war the patient with the hysterical paralysis was complacent so long as he thought he was honourably retiring from the struggle, but it was surprising how often one found that this apparent complacency was only a semi-conscious effort at self-deception and how often the patient had an inner feeling that things were not quite right. In industrial conditions, hysterical paralysis and other symptoms are not uncommon, and the patient is often genuinely anxious to get rid of them, although they may have been initiated in connexion with an impulse to avoid work. However, he is trying to recover in the wrong way, perhaps by further straining instead of by relaxation, and will not succeed until he is shown by the physician how to get out of his difficulty, and is led back to an adequate adjustment to life.

If then the neurotic needs a physician, if he cannot, of his own unaided effort, regain his adjustment, who is to be that physician? Let it be stated at once, that no individual, however skilled and however eminent, can hope to succeed with every neurotic. Every neurotic personality is different from his neighbour, the personality of every physician is different from that of any other, and it stands to reason that if A B C are any neurotics and X Y Z any physicians, X may find he can help A and B, but not C, while Y may help B and C, but not A, and so on. Next, need the word physician, as used here, be translated literally to mean a medical man? Theoretically, no; a priest, a schoolmaster, or any man or woman of affairs might do. But as a matter of practical politics, it is doubtful if anyone but the medical man can, by reason of his training, adequately comprehend the whole personality of the neurotic, his body and mind and his whole relation to his environment, and if any of these are neglected the cure of the neurosis is apt to be but a haphazard and imperfect affair. Clearly even every medical man cannot hope to deal successfully with the more seriously afflicted neurotic. At present at all events, it must be the special field of the medical psychologist, who requires very special training and aptitude for the work, and must go on learning and improving his understanding all his life. Whoever the physician may be, he must not lose sight of the necessity to take a comprehensive view of the whole personality of his patient and therefore he must never be biased or a faddist. This unfortunately is what so many lay psychotherapists are apt to be. With all respect to the claim of the Church to the efficacy of spiritual healing, the weak point of such a method is, that its point of attack must be to induce an emotional religious experience, to use James' term. This may and does remove symptoms and in many cases the removal of symptoms is all that is required to enable the patient to readjust himself towards life, at any rate for the time being. None the less this form of healing can never be universally successful even in neurosis, because it cannot take sufficient account of the bodily needs, if the vicious circle has gone too far, and because it does not take account of the frequent need for intellectual enlightenment and emotional adjustment, apart from simple suggestion, which are essential before a cure can be obtained.

Next, the physician, whoever he may be, must abjure all tendency to judge and only seek to understand. Judgments, rewards and punishments are essential for society, and are applicable to the individual in relation to society, but are much less useful for the individual in relationship to himself or to another single individual. The schoolmaster who finds the small boy corrupting other small boys must punish the one in order to protect the many, and the policeman who finds

Bill Sikes stealing his neighbour's cash-box must hale him before the judge, who must inflict punishment lest Bill Sikes goes and does likewise to his other neighbours. But this is not the business of the physician. He must ask, " Why did he do this ? " and the answer is frequently surprisingly obvious. How often does the patient in a state of trembling agitation say : " Doctor, I can't tell you this. I don't know what you will think of me, you will never speak to me again,"—and when with great trepidation he does relate the experience to the physician and finds that the latter is not in the least moved to horror or reproach, the patient is not only surprised, but enormously relieved and encouraged. Whatever the experience is, the physician must not even think, much less say : " How disgusting !" " How dreadful ! " " How revolting ! " He must simply ask : " Why did this thing happen ? What were the factors in the patient's ego and his environment, which determined just this pattern of behaviour ? " As has been said, it frequently happens that, looked at unemotionally, these determinants are obvious and the explanation to the patient establishes and cements the confidence in the physician, which is so necessary for a cure. The physician must eschew judgments and strive for understanding, and he must have sympathy for his patient however poor a thing he may appear to be, remembering that he is trying to recover and needs help. It is probably impossible for anyone to feel sympathy with every one, and if the physician finds that he does not sympathize with any given patient, he ought not to treat that patient. It means that he is up against one of those incompatibilities between personalities, which had better be recognized sooner rather than later, as an attempt at too close contact is likely to make for harm rather than good. This sympathy of the physician for his patient must not be of the passive sort, but essentially active. He must really desire to help his patient and be prepared to take all pains to that

Q

end. He must be ready to take infinite trouble himself, and must, if occasion demands, be willing to subject his patient to considerable discomfort and distress if he is convinced that ultimate good will ensue. Just as the surgeon does not shrink from inflicting physical pain, if that is the only means whereby the patient can be restored to health, so the psychotherapist must be willing to subject his patient to mental pain if this is necessary for his salvation. Freud has stated that no one ought to undertake psychoanalysis unless he himself has been fully analysed. If the view is accepted that Freudian analysis is the only way in which self-knowledge and self-control may be obtained, then this contention is right, for no one who deceives himself or is not in control of his emotional reactions will succeed in the treatment of the neurotic. However, I personally am not convinced that all who have been analysed have necessarily reached that desirable state, nor that those who have not been analysed are incapable of reaching a sufficient degree of self-knowledge and self-control. Therefore, I do not share the opinion that every psychotherapist should be analysed, but I do believe it is very necessary for him to be honest with himself and to recognize his limitations. This is specially the case with regard to sex, for as we have seen, he will have to do with sex in many of his patients, and the management of the relationship between physician and patient is one of the most difficult of all the many phases of psychotherapy, but he must also control his temper—not always an easy task—for neurotics can be, beyond words, exasperating. I believe that if a good relationship is established, it may do no harm and perhaps good, for the physician thoroughly to lose his temper with the patient once, but this is essentially an exception which proves the rule and certainly should never be practised deliberately. Endless patience, perseverance and equanimity must be the rôle of the physician in the face of all backslidings and perversities. Many a patient has been literally driven back to adjustment and good health by the unfailing good temper and perseverance of his physician. Sometimes it appears as though the patient were deliberately trying to provoke the latter, but the wise physician knows that this is not really so, it is only one part of the patient's personality—that the patterns which comprise the impulses resisting adaptation have, for the time being, gained ascendancy. It must be remembered that there is good in every neurotic, and it is the duty of the physician to find that good and stick to it through thick and thin. If he cannot find the good he ought to hand over the patient to someone who can. Every neurotic has a sense of inferiority, whether obvious or hidden, since his failure of adaptation necessarily leads to this, and he must find someone who believes in him through everything.

The Freudian school has laid very special stress on the relationship between physician and patient, and has called this relationship " transference." [1] They regard it as the most important single factor in psychotherapy, insisting that without transference nothing can be accomplished, but, given a well-managed transference, even the worst case can always be helped if not cured.

By transference we mean that bond which binds patient to physician during the treatment. What this bond is, it is very difficult to define. According to the Freudians, the term has a definite sexual connotation. The physician stands to the patient in the rôle of father substitute, a situation, which, in their concept, involves real sexual attraction with the ambivalent emotional reaction of excessive dependence on the one hand or jealous hatred on the other. These reactions give rise to positive and negative transference, which may make their appearance alternately in the same course of treatment. As we find to be very generally the case with Freudian concepts when divested of their crudities, there is a great deal of

[1] S. Freud. Collected Papers II, p. 312. London 1924.

truth in this description of the special relatedness of physician to patient as enunciated by Freud. It cannot be expected, however, that the general public should trouble to sift the grain from the chaff in this or any other Freudian "pronunciamento." Therefore they accept it at its face value, and believe that psychotherapy involves the situation in which the patient must definitely fall in love with the physician. This, perhaps naturally, is an objectionable and dangerous state of affairs in the eyes of the public in general and the relations of the patient in particular, and explains to a certain extent the antagonism toward psychotherapy exhibited by so many people. This, however, is not all, for in whatever way we look at it, it is clear that the patient is dependent on and attached to the physician in a quite peculiar way. Firstly the physician is a "medicine-man" to the patient, using the term to imply the priest-doctor conception of the primitive. As doctor he guards and understands the physical needs and cures the bodily aches and pains of the patient ; this needs no elaboration, and is readily accepted by both the patient and his friends. As priest he ministers to the spiritual needs of the patient. A contemporary man of letters is credited with the aphorism, that psychoanalysis represents all the tortures of the confessional without the grace of absolution. The first phrase is doubtless correct, for the patient is frequently called upon to confess his manifold sins and wickedness, but I am not so sure that the second phrase holds good. For those who believe that the only possible absolution is that which is delivered by the authority and through the ministrations of the Church no doubt help should be sought through the orthodox channels of their religion, but even for those, and certainly for countless others, an understanding of the impulses, which led up to the particular pattern of behaviour, is of immense help, and it is in the rôle of the exponent of these determinants of behaviour that the physician must take on himself the duties of priest.

After all, it is easy to blame the Old Gentleman for all our lapses from virtue, but it is not until we realize that the personality of His Satanic Majesty emerges from our own primitive and uncontrolled impulses, that we can do much to better our condition. To understand why we committed a fault is not necessarily to condone it, but rather to take better care and exercise greater control lest we fall into the same ditch in the future. The neurotic is all too apt to wallow in the slough of his past delinquencies, real or imaginary, and it is only when we rouse him from this and force him to look to the future, and not to the past, that we begin to put him on the path to health. He must learn the lesson that Maeterlinck taught,[1] that a man's past is within his control and, if he uses it to drag him back into remorse, he is damned, but if he uses it as a spur to fresh and better endeavour in the future, he is blessed. I have no knowledge of how this may work in Catholic communities, but in Protestant circles this relationship presents special difficulties, with regard to both the patient and his friends. The patient, if of an independent type, may resent submitting himself to the direction of the physician and may fear to give his soul too much into the keeping of another, just because he so much feels the need of doing so. His relatives and friends have seemed almost impossibly obtuse in their failure to understand his difficulties, and need of sympathy, and when the patient finds someone who is able to understand, he is afraid of going to the opposite extreme and losing the " command of his soul " altogether. The relatives still more resent the priest relationship, because they are really concerned to help the patient and cannot understand why they are not able to do so. The physician may quite rightly explain to the patient that his relatives cannot understand him for want of the requisite knowledge, and therefore cannot help him. Too often it is then reported to the

[1] M. Maeterlinck, " The Past " *Fortnightly Review*, March 1901.

relatives that the doctor said: " You do not, and you don't even want to understand me and help me," a statement which is naturally resented.   However, there is more in transference than the medicine-man relationship.   In every personality of whichever sex, there is both a masculine and feminine element and the physician takes on the position of father substitute towards the masculine element and represents the ideal of chivalry for the feminine element.   The patient will regard him as the father is regarded by the growing boy. He is someone dependable, someone who is always there when wanted, ready to help out of a scrape but not to be trifled with.   He knows a great deal—perhaps everything—his judgment is dependable and can always be referred to with confidence.   He holds up an ideal which should be followed with all the effort that is possible, and he points out the path to manhood and health.   But the patient will also regard him, when transference is complete, as a woman often regards a man who is stronger and wiser than herself, as rather a hero, as someone with infinite compassion and understanding, one who will stand by her through thick and thin.   It is this relationship which calls for such tact and care on the part of the physician, such self-knowledge and self-control. Theoretically it may be said that this last relationship is unnecessary, but practically it is a relationship which does frequently occur, and in view of the childishness of the neurotic cannot be easily avoided.   Nor should the risk be minimized ; after all we are all human, and perfect control is an attribute of deity and not of humanity, and cases do occur when moral and social disaster ensue, but this is a risk which must be run if successful treatment of neurosis is to take place, just as the risk of infection and death must be taken in any medical practice, nor is this risk by any means confined to psychotherapy.   However, as a matter of usual practice, it is not so bad as all this ; we have described the attitude of the patient to the physician in transference, but this is not the attitude of the physician to his patient. The neurotic patient is presented, or should be presented to the physician, as, on the one hand a child who needs help, and on the other an intellectual problem clamouring for a solution. So long as the physician is fairly balanced and honest with himself, and not the subject of unhealthy repressions in respect of his sex impulse, he is not likely to run off the rails either with a child or with an intellectual problem. Moreover, we must never forget that the attitude of the neurotic is childish, and is not specially dangerous if the physician plays his part and realizes that he has special responsibilities to face in respect to transference. It would probably be as well that the facts of transference should be clearly explained both to the patient and, if possible, to the relatives, though it often happens that the patient consults the psychotherapist in direct opposition to the wishes of his relations. In this case, provided that the patient is of age and legally responsible, the physician is perfectly right in consenting to treat him, and the relations must be placated as occasion arises. In all cases help might be obtained by the extension of what might be called consolatory consultations, where another physician is called in, not to investigate the case or alter treatment, which would be impossible at one interview, but to reassure both patient and relatives that the right thing is being done. This consultant might be specially useful in explaining the nature and peculiarities of transference, and allaying the natural qualms felt on this subject by all concerned.

But as has been said the physician should not have any real difficulty in managing the transference. He must take charge of the whole situation to begin with, and gradually, as the patient begins to be able to make adjustments, he must retire more and more into the background, until the latter stands entirely on his or her own feet. Some patients never

reach this stage and the physician must maintain some degree
of transference, the directorship of Janet, for an indefinite
time, and this often calls for the most careful judgment. The
friends may think that he is assuming too great an ascendancy
over the patient, they may even calumniate him abominably,
but the physician must be honest with himself; he must of
course avoid any tendency to keep the rôle of director for his
own advantage, but if he really believes that his patient
requires him and cannot do without him, it is his duty to
stick by that patient whatever happens.

Transference may break down in two ways. Either it
outruns the constable and a too close emotional and even
physical attraction springs up between the physician and the
patient. This risk has already been referred to, and if the
physician recognizes it, he ought to break off treatment,
at any rate for the time. On the other hand a negative transference may be established which becomes unmanageable.
By negative transference is meant the establishment of a
repulsion towards the physician, so that the patient resists
his help, showing his dislike by inflicting on him personal
annoyances, ranging from failure to keep his appointments
to malignant libel. This represents the activity of that pattern
of impulses which resist readjustment and are frequently
exhibited by insane persons, but much less frequently by
neurotics. It may be a transitory phase, comparable to a fit of
naughtiness in a small boy, who will not obey his father, or
it may be much more permanent. If so, the physician must
realize that he is not the personality to find and encourage
the good elements in his patient, but must hand him over to
someone else who may be more successful. It is evident therefore that the successful treatment of the neurotic calls for the
exhibition of all that is best in the physician, and although
the work is hard and the knowledge required encyclopædic,
the problems are of great interest and the help which can be

given is enormous, for the neurotic patient really does suffer more than most people realize. Apart from this, however, the physician in treating the neurotic has an opportunity to develop his own personality and understanding, which no other activity can give him to the same extent, and this is its own reward.

CHAPTER XIII

BODY AND MIND IN THE TREATMENT OF NEUROSIS

In the distant past it was the fashion to regard neurotic symptoms as manifestations of purely physical ailments, thus hysteria, as its name implies, was thought to be due to a derangement of the womb and so forth. Later it was recognized, that while there was no structural alteration manifest in the various organs, such as could be demonstrated at post-mortem examinations, their function was deranged in some subtle way. This was a decided advance in the understanding of neurosis, but it was still contended that the cause of this derangement of function was physical and bodily, due to alimentary poisons, bacillary toxins and the rest. Then, under the influence of Charcot and his pupils Freud and Janet, who attacked the subject from widely different angles, the psychogenic influences were brought into prominence, and this school of thought has gradually gained ground in the last twenty-five years. After the failure of Mott in the early stages of the war to prove that the manifestations of " shell shock " were due to petechial hæmorrhages in the central nervous system, and the conversion of this great pathologist to the psychogenic theory, the latter may be said to have swept the board for a time and, as was perhaps natural, the pendulum undoubtedly swung too far and neurotic symptoms were described exclusively in terms of psychic derangement, and the bodily factor was in many cases lost sight of altogether. After the war the increasing knowledge about the endocrine system diverted attention from the purely psychogenic concept to theories attributing neurotic derangements to disturbances in the balance of these secretions. There were some who, still fain to cling to the physical explanations, welcomed these researches as after all justifying their contentions that bodily rather than mental factors had to be taken into account if the neurotic symptoms were to be explained.

The controversies which have raged among the various schools of thought have undoubtedly originated in and owed much of their bitterness to the age-long conflict between idealists and realists, between animists and materialists and perhaps between theologians and evolutionists. The modern developments of physics and biology, however, have clearly indicated that the distinction between spirit and matter and between mind and body is more apparent than real.

Huxley's contention that there is no psychosis without a neurosis,[1] and conversely Lloyd Morgan's suggestion that there is no physical process in life without a mental aspect,[2] are certainly helpful in dealing with the neurotic, and it would be well if they could be recognized more widely. The first premise implies that whenever a mental process is experienced by the patient a certain pattern of neurones is activated, and as Semon has pointed out there can be no activation of such patterns without some modification of their structures occurring, however infinitesimal this may be. Furthermore, we know that no pattern of neurones can be activated in isolation, that is to say that the activation tends to spread through other neurones. This means that as a direct sequence of what appears to be a purely mental process not only may modifications be induced in the central nervous system, but, as a result of the spread of activation from the original pattern, definite bodily changes,

[1] T. H. Huxley, *Essays.* London 1893–4.
[2] C. Lloyd Morgan, *Emergent Evolution.* London 1923.

such as contraction of muscles, secretion of glands and so on, may take place.

The second premise implies that no bodily activity can take place, without some sort of mental accompaniment, though this latter may be quite below the level of consciousness, and so the subject may be completely unaware of it. However we know that unconscious mental processes may profoundly influence the activity of the conscious level and also by the spread of activity, patterns may be brought into play whose mental aspects enjoy consciousness. We must keep clearly before us therefore both the mental and physical processes which occur in the course of the illness, and try to estimate their relative importance and their true origin. We have adopted as our principle that neurosis is caused by the failure of adaptation within the personality. Further, we have contended that it is only at the level of deity that complete harmony and perfect adaptation can pertain. At the level of humanity, circumstances may arise in any personality which may cause a breakdown and such a lowering of that compromise which we regard as normal adaptation, that the individual must be considered to be " out of health." In other words, anyone may theoretically become neurotic if there is sufficient increase in the difficulty of circumstances or lowering of his power to deal with them. The war illustrated this admirably : circumstances certainly became more difficult, and comparatively strong, healthy people, who had no difficulty in adjustment to civil conditions of life, broke down. At the same time these breakdowns were more frequent under the stress of certain mental factors on the one hand and of certain physical factors on the other. Endopsychic conflict is itself a failure of adaptation and therefore if sufficiently severe must induce pathological symptoms, but, in so far as perfect adaptation is impossible, we must, even in health, achieve sufficient adaptation at the expense of overcoming

frictions by an extra expenditure of energy. If one may use
the comparison with due apology to that great man, Mr Henry
Ford, we are like his car which overcomes the imperfectly
adjusted fittings by the high horse-power developed. It
follows therefore that if anything occurs to lower our horse-
power our machine will not go and our adaptation breaks down.
Such causes may be entirely physical, and that is why such
illnesses as influenza, pneumonia and typhoid, and such
physical accidents as loss of blood or deprivation of proper
food so often seem to determine a nervous breakdown. In
some cases the recovery of physical strength is sufficient
and the machine can again overcome its frictions, but too
often a vicious circle has been set up, whereby the friction has
meantime increased so that the ordinary horse-power of the
engine cannot overcome it and allow the personality to achieve
sufficient adaptation. Similarly, in psychogenic cases, we find
that in the course of the illness the physical health has
suffered to such an extent that unless this receives attention
no recovery can result. The truth is that wherever the failure
of adaptation occurs within the personality there is a reper-
cussion through the whole, and no part of it escapes some
derangement. As a result we find that function is upset in all
parts of the body, partly as the result of the poisons of fatigue
and partly as the result of disturbance of the balance of the
endocrine glands and the vegetative nervous system. It is
generally conceded that structure is not affected in neurotic
illness, but we ought not to be too dogmatic on this point
if the maladjustment lasts long enough. No one will deny that
prolonged anxiety will produce abnormalities in gastric
secretion and vascular distribution. Abnormalities in secretion
and vascular distribution may be responsible for all sorts of
structural changes. Again prolonged disturbances in the
endocrine balance may determine arterio-sclerotic changes
which may eventually be responsible for cerebral hæmorrhage,

and so on. Moreover we must not shut our eyes to the fact that neurotic illness undoubtedly renders the patient less resistant to infection, with all its potentialities for destruction of structure. For these reasons we might tentatively accept the doctrine that deity—that is a state of perfect adjustment to environment—will know no illness and perhaps no death, for if there were never any maladjustments there would be no structural change. This is the rock on which Christian Science founders, for this doctrine presumes that the quality of Deity has already been attained. However, all that is mere speculation, and for practical purposes we may say that neurosis does not produce structural change, and therefore should be capable of complete cure, if due regard is given to the whole personality of the patient.

As has been said, functional derangement is induced by fatigue and by interference with the balance of the endocrine and vegetative nervous systems. We have seen that failure of adaptation results in conflict, that conflict results in resistances, dissociations and friction, and these mean increased work and fatigue. Fatigue is the expression of the toxic effects of the waste products incident to work done—the ashes of the fire. These " ashes " are definitely poisonous, and the poisons are absorbed into the blood and lymph streams, as well as being dumped at the seat of the performance of the work.

Organs which are perfused with blood containing poisons will not function efficiently, and so a vicious circle is set up, for the inefficiency of the vital organs results in greater liability to fatigue and the production of further poisons. One of the most important systems to be deranged is that of the endocrine organs, though whether these are directly affected by emotional conflict or through the intervention of fatigue products cannot be determined with certainty. Such upset in turn is apt to disturb the function of all organs but more especially that of the vegetative nervous system and the balance between sympathetic and parasympathetic activity. Again, it is doubtful if this is influenced directly by the conflict or only through the interventions of the endocrine disturbances. Once vegetative nervous activity is upset, however, all sorts of functional derangements may ensue, as this determines the regulation of blood supply to the various parts of the body, of the secretions of the various glands, and the state of tension of at least the involuntary muscles, while its influence in determining pain and alterations in postural tone in the voluntary muscles is only now beginning to be investigated.

A very important bodily factor in determining the location of neurotic symptoms is what Adler has called organ inferiority. By this he means that some organ or part of the body has been more weakly than the rest, so that it is more liable to injuries or disease, whether gross or insignificant. In many cases this is fairly obvious : we are all acquainted with the life-long dyspeptic, with the lady who suffers from " mucous colitis " for years and years, or in other words who has a sluggish colon and so suffers from constipation. Since the muscles cannot cope with the impaction the attempt is made more or less successfully to overcome this by extra lubrication, hence the mucus, and the complete absence of true colitis which characterizes these patients. In other cases the inferiority is less obvious, but the frequency with which one limb is subject to minor injuries as compared to the others is suggestive of inferiority. As Adie [1] has pointed out in relation to " functional " disturbances of the central nervous system, careful observation will usually disclose cases of undoubted structural defect exhibiting the same symptoms. This enables us to " localize " the functional derangement ; and at any rate in some cases this " locality " is probably a " locus inferior."

There is no question that hysterical symptoms are often associated with inferior organs, and the very inferiority acts

[1] W. J. Adie, *Brain* III., 1926.

as a suggestion towards disability. It is an interesting subject for discussion why inferiority of organs occurs and whether this is congenital or acquired. For example, a lady had a severe pelvic neurosis associated with a marked sexual repression dating from experiences at the age of five or six. She had an infantile uterus and a varicose condition of all three orifices which constituted a definite organ inferiority. This varicose condition was closely associated with her physical discomforts, and may quite well have been connected with a lack of balance of the sympathetic and parasympathetic control through her pelvic plexus. But to what extent this imbalance and the infantile condition of the uterus were the result of the mental repressions and emotional conflicts, and to what extent they were strictly congenital, cannot be determined.

Since neurotic patients generally come to us with the vicious circle fully developed, in which mind acts on body and body on mind, theoretical discussion, resembling that on the primogeniture of the hen and the egg, is of no practical use. What is of use however, is the consideration of how we are to attack the vicious circle. In this respect people are apt to exhibit intellectual snobbishness of the worst descrip-tion. Those who hold with the psychogenic causation of neurosis are apt to regard the administration of drugs as something reprehensible, while the endocrine enthusiasts regard any attempt at mental healing as a waste of time. For example I remember a friend who did not believe in psycho-therapy asking me in a voice vibrating with scorn what I thought of a man who put a patient to sleep by hypnosis but had given him a dose of bromide first. Why on earth shouldn't he do this? If the bromide was needed to quieten the patient sufficiently to make hypnosis possible, and if hypnosis was effective, so that stronger and more dangerous hypnotics were unnecessary, the combination of the two therapeutic agents seems to be very good practice. If a neurotic patient is to recover, he must first get encouragement and confidence in his physician, and if the physician can remove or relieve a distressing symptom by the administration of drugs, he will achieve both purposes, even if the remedy is merely symptomatic and the symptom of small consequence in relation to the whole breakdown. Further, we must pay attention to the patient's subjective symptoms and not dismiss them as imaginary. If a patient complains of pain it may be taken that he is experiencing that pain. Pain cannot be imagined. Either the patient is telling a deliberate lie and is malingering, which is rare, or he is actually suffering as he says. If he is suffering it is our duty to discover whether there is an adequate physical stimulus, which we reckon would produce such pain in anyone, or whether the patient is over-sensitive and responding unduly to an insignificant stimulus. If a patient experiences the prick of a pin as if it was the thrust of a sword we may justly say he is over-sensitive, but we must remember that over-sensitivity is a symptom which must be removed, generally by mental means. This most people will admit, but they do not always remember that it is not a bad thing to remove the pin, even if it is not a sword, and this attention to small bodily ailments is quite frequently an essential to success in treatment. Care must of course be taken to approach such small ailments in the right way, so as to avoid fixing the attention of the patient still further on the minor ailments of the body, but, because such should not be stressed, it does not mean that they should be totally neglected. During a course of treatment it is not difficult for the experienced physician to determine on what days he should confine himself to purely mental treatment and when he may give his attention to the removal of these lesser physical pin pricks. The administration of drugs is not only a legitimate but in some cases an essential part of the treatment, but the success of a drug must not blind

R

the physician to its significance. In the milder cases a tonic
in one instance or a sedative in another is sometimes successful in restoring the horse-power in relation to the friction, to
return to our previous analogy, and adaptation is restored.
This success is apt to establish various remedies as specifics
for the cure of " neurasthenia," but too often the more severely
afflicted patient tries such remedies one after the other, only
to find that although according to the testimonials, they have
cured every other patient, they don't cure him, and he gets
more depressed and more convinced that his illness is unique,
that no one has ever been afflicted as he is afflicted and that
no one can possibly cure him. None the less such remedies
are useful, especially phosphorus compounds and lecithin
as tonics, and valerian and bromide preparations as sedatives,
but none of them are specifics for neurosis. There never has
been, never will be, and never can be a specific for neurosis,
for every case is a separate problem, a vicious circle started
by a failure of adaptation, and only to be resolved by a restoration of that adaptation. Drugs are too apt to be empirical
remedies—bottle No. I for those with cough, bottle No. II
for headache, and so on, and in no class of illness can such
methods of treatment be so futile and detrimental as in neurosis.
However, drugs and physical methods of treatment, such as
massage and electricity, have their place so long as the physician
knows exactly what he is doing and why he is using them,
but when one meets a masseuse who tells one that she cures
all neurasthenics with high frequency, one makes a mental
note never on any account to send her a patient. In long-
standing cases, the bodily symptoms may be very difficult to
cure, since a habit has arisen, which has sunk below the level
at which conscious control is possible,—for example, the young
girl, to whom we have already referred, who suffered from a
tic, in which her head was turned to one side with a contortion
of the facial muscles expressing a most lively disgust. This

at times was magnified into a general convulsive attack, which was diagnosed as epileptic. A very short period of observation was sufficient to establish the fact that the attacks were hysterical and not epileptic. Further mental exploration disclosed that both the head-turning tic and the generalized convulsions were hysterical symptoms in association with marked sexual repressions, established during the middle period of adolescence, and that there was a good deal of mental disturbance in this connexion as well, which continued in the intervals between attacks and expressed itself in anxieties and nightmares. It was possible to resolve these conflicts, at any rate to a very large extent, and the general attacks entirely ceased, all anxiety and dreams disappeared, and the tic was reduced in frequency and severity except during the monthly periods which were painful and prolonged. The tic was certainly a low-level habit, and yet its association with the period suggested that it was still conditioned by sex. No doubt the Freudian analyst would contend that the treatment was too superficial and that the tic and perhaps the dysmenorrhea would disappear if more deeply lying conflicts were unmasked. This might be so, but circumstances were such that the further probing of the sex life seemed undesirable, especially as the remaining symptom was in no way disabling and only mildly annoying to the patient. On the other hand all tics are not psychogenic in origin, for example, cases of spasmodic torticollis seem to be due to an uncontrolled activity of a reflex arc involving the nuclei situated in the hind-brain. The above case may be of a similar nature and in such a case it is doubtful if the most complete analysis could induce an establishment of control over this arc. In such a case, if there were any physical means of stopping the activity of this arc, which unfortunately is not so, they ought unhesitatingly to be used, and I have no doubt whatever that the removal of this last symptom by such means would complete the cure. It behoves us, therefore, to be very much on our guard against any intellectual snobbishness, or narrowness of vision, and to use any weapon which is useful, in our efforts to break the vicious circle of a neurosis at any or every point, but at the same time we ought to be quite sure, why we are using the weapon, and if it proves useful, determine exactly why it has done so, and how much or how little it has accomplished.

To sum up this argument, we believe that neurosis in the great majority of cases is of mental origin and must be treated by psychotherapy, but if it is prolonged, the mental causative agents and the resulting disturbance of the central nervous system may result in physical symptoms. These physical symptoms may become very troublesome to the patient, and if they can be relieved or removed by physical means, the physician should not hesitate to use such means.

CHAPTER XIV

THE SCOPE AND LIMITATIONS OF PSYCHOANALYSIS

A VAST literature has grown up around psychoanalysis ; several periodicals have been devoted entirely to its exposition, but still there is a remarkable confusion of thought as to its value and desirability. During the period after the war, when those who had done the work of that strenuous time were glad of a rest from the somewhat over-sensational happenings of the previous four years, the common herd of sensational extraverts found the absence of their daily lurid thrills tedious and depressing. Unfortunately some of these people discovered that " psychoanalysis," a procedure about as much divorced from real psychoanalysis as anything could possibly be, gave them all the thrills they needed, and not to have been " psychoed " became as *démodée* as not to have been shingled became three or four years later. As the reputable practitioners persisted in treating the matter seriously and neither gave the thrills or revelations which were required, the demand created the supply of unorthodox practitioners who were merely purveyors of pornography. This gave rise to a natural but ill-merited wholesale condemnation of the process, and to the demands of terrified " Disgusteds " and " Paterfamiliases " in the daily press for enquiries and even legal suppression of all those who professed to have anything to do with this form of black magic. The National Council for Mental Hygiene and the Representative Body of the British Medical Association both undertook enquiries for the purpose of furnishing reports at the instigation of responsible members of the medical profession and the lay public who really wanted guidance on this vexed question. That such a report could be produced was a matter for grave doubt amongst many experienced officials of both societies, for the truth is that the subject has got itself into great confusion both as to what it really is and what it really achieves. As to the latter question, it may be that sufficient time has not yet elapsed, since its practice became widespread and much developed, to afford real proof as to its efficacy, and the whole question is still in the stage when it is a more fitting subject for technical debate than for formal report. These considerations would seem to give more than adequate grounds for not proceeding further with this chapter, and yet I believe the issue should not be shirked, for it may be easier to present an individual opinion than a formal report, since the former is of relatively little importance and only carries the weight of its intrinsic value, whereas a formal report is a much more serious matter and demands, if it does not command, the respect of those who have requested its presentation.

It is necessary to consider what psychoanalysis is, but first it may be as well to dismiss certain misconceptions. In the first place psychoanalysis is not a sort of glorified history-taking, in which great and sometimes irrelevant detail is obtained from the patient by the ordinary methods practised by the careful physician since medicine began. Detailed anamnesis is certainly a necessary preliminary to the treatment of the neurotic, but it is not psychoanalysis, which aims at the discovery and disentanglement of impulses and parts of the personality of which the patient is unaware. In the second place psychoanalysis is not a didactic series of suggestions as to the management of the patient's conscious sexual life either in accordance with, or in opposition to the social code. I have heard the implication that both these represented the activities of psychoanalysis from practically the same source in the same afternoon.

Psychoanalysis was a term coined by Sigmund Freud to describe a special method of treatment applied to neurotic patients. He himself in 1909 attributed its origin to Breuer, but rightly repudiated this five years later, claiming psychoanalysis as his own and Breuer's cathartic method as its precursor.[1] For this reason Freud and his immediate disciples seem perfectly justified in asserting that their special technique is the only true psychoanalysis. None the less since the general public has come to regard the methods of such psychotherapists as Jung and Adler as psychoanalysis, reference to their modifications of the original method must be made.

The story of the origin and development of psychoanalysis has been told over and over again and can only be briefly referred to here. In the year 1880, the Viennese physician Breuer was treating a case of hysteria by hypnosis. While in a hypnotic trance, the patient related a long train of events, some of which had occurred far back in her childhood. The narration was accompanied by marked emotional excitement, and after the patient was restored to full consciousness, her general condition was considerably improved. Following the suggestion offered on this occasion Breuer and Freud investigated the effect of what they called abreaction.[2] This they describe as the freeing of " confined affect," which occurs when the patient is induced to relate an experience which was originally accompanied by considerable affective reaction, and which has not been allowed to come into consciousness for some considerable time. What really happens is that the engram, which subserves the set of ideas relating to the experience, is reassociated, so that it achieves that relatedness which involves consciousness. So, from the psychological aspect,

---

[1] S. Freud, *Collected Papers*, I, p. 288. London 1925.
[2] Breuer and Freud, *Studien über Hysterie*. Vienna 1895

the experience is reintegrated with proper relation to time and space, and in proper proportion to the rest of the personality. It is this reintegration which induces the therapeutic benefit, and not the mere ebullition of emotional excitement. This relief by "abreaction" is familiar in present-day psycho-therapy, but its investigators soon found that abreaction in itself was not enough, in many cases of neurosis. Freud thereupon turned his attention away from pure therapeutics, and initiated an enquiry into the mental processes of neurotics. Even so recently as 1920 he remarks: "At the present time theoretical knowledge is still far more important to all of us than therapeutic success." [1]

In order to get at the forgotten memories whose revival with abreaction was so beneficial to the patient, Freud introduced the method of free association. The patient having been placed in a completely relaxed state is encouraged to allow a "chain of associations" to pass through his mind, without guidance or selection by conscious effort. The result sooner or later is either that the patient comes to a full stop when he encounters a resistance imposed as the result of conflict, which has been discussed in Chapter II, or a memory is revived with more or less abreaction. In this process it is the duty of the physician to be a passive observer of the train of associations, noting and recording resistances and abreactions and perhaps assisting the patient to correlate and understand the implications of these. However, free association alone was a confusing and laborious proceeding, and attention had soon to be turned to the simplification and shortening of the method of investigation. This led to the study of dreams which pointed the way to the theories of repression, resistance and infantile sexuality, which have already been discussed. Dreams were, according to Freud, indirect expressions of repressed complexes, distorted and modified in the process of

---

[1] S. Freud, *International Journal of Psychoanalysis*, 1920.

conflict. They were then the royal road to the unconscious and became important matter for investigation and interpretion in the course of treatment, since the unmasking of these unconscious complexes was the avowed object of the analyst. Having got so far it became obvious that from the therapeutic standpoint there were two salient features which were met with in dealing with any patient. The first was that the relationship between patient and physician was different, at least in intensity, from that established in the treatment of other diseases, and that a study of this transference threw considerable light on the patient's unconscious emotional attitudes towards those nearest to him in life. It was maintained by Freud that in the course of transference the physician became a substitute for father, mother, husband, wife, etc., as the case might be. The second was that certain promising lines of enquiry were cut short by resistances which could only be overcome with great difficulty and by devious methods. Moreover, it was maintained that it was only by a study of these resistances, their origin and nature, that a true insight into the conflicts of the patient could be obtained. So important does Freud consider these two features of psychoanalysis that he says: "Any line of investigation, no matter what its direction, which recognizes these two facts and takes them as the starting-point of its work, may call itself psychoanalysis, though it arrives at results other than my own. But anyone who takes up other sides of the problem, while avoiding these two premises, will hardly escape the charge of mis-appropriating by attempted impersonation, if he persists in calling himself a psychoanalyst." [1]

The study of dreams naturally led to the question, How does "the censor" distort the latent content of the dream, so as to convert it into the manifest content? The answer to this was that it is done by symbolization, and it was remarked

[1] S. Freud, *Collected Papers*, I, p. 298. London 1925.

that many dream symbols corresponded, or seemed to correspond, to the symbols familiar in folk-lore and in the normal customs of primitive man. This gave rise to the theory of the universality of symbols and presented a further short cut in treatment. If certain symbols had a fixed value, there was no necessity to waste time while the patient found out the meaning of these symbols for himself; they could be interpreted by the physician, and this interpretation would start the patient off on the right path to overcome resistance and disclose the hidden complex. Having come to the conclusion empirically that all neuroses were of sexual origin, it followed that all symbols were sexual, and so an alarming list of convex objects occurring in dreams were held to be symbols of the male organ, while a similar list of concave or hollow objects were regarded as symbolic of the female genitals. With the development of the study of symbols psychoanalysis came to be applied in many fields outside medicine—in literature, art, and philosophy, but these excursions do not concern us here, and, interesting as they are, must not tempt us from the study of neurosis.

After the study and classification of symbols came the attempt to classify resistances, again an effort to make short cuts in treatment. For example, Freud suggests: "In male patients the most important resistances to the treatment seem to be derived from the father complex and to express themselves in fear of the father and in defiance and incredulity towards him." [1] Since in the course of transference the physician so often becomes a father substitute, this resistance is of considerable importance, if common, and it certainly is. Just as the patient develops transference towards the physician, so the physician may develop transference towards the patient, and in order to control this and prevent untoward results, the doctrine came to be laid down that the physician must

[1] S. Freud, *Collected Papers*, I, p. 288. London 1925.

either analyse himself or be analysed. It may be agreed at once that it is indeed necessary for the physician who is dealing with neurotics to have insight into and control of his emotional reactions, but as has been said before, it is doubtful if analysis is essential.

In addition to the memories of the patients, which come up during the course of an analysis, the physician must closely observe the behaviour of the patient, since in this behaviour he repeats infantile attitudes which give a clue to the repressed material. It is often found that, when the resistances are so great that no recollections can come up, these repetitions in behaviour are more than usually manifest and await the interpretation of the observant physician. For example, the phenomenon which frequently occurs in transference, that of the woman patient falling in love with her physician, does not represent a " conquest " by the physician but a repetition of infantile fixations, and the situation may be used by the physician who knows what he is about, to explore these and get them into consciousness and control, so that the patient may be freed from them for the future.

It has been urged by some that after analysis must come synthesis, but this apparently logical demand certainly obscures the meaning and effect of psychoanalysis. It seems worth while to quote Freud on this point : [1] " The neurotic human being brings us his mind racked and rent by resistances. Whilst we are working at analysis of it and at removing the resistances, this mind of his begins to grow together ; that great unity which we call his ego fuses into one all the instinctive trends, which before had been split off and barred away from it. The psycho-synthesis is thus achieved during analytic treatment without intervention, automatically and inevitably. We have created the conditions for it by dissolving the symptoms into their elements and by removing the resistances.

---

[1] S. Freud, *Collected Papers*, II, p. 295. London 1925.

There is no truth in the idea that when the patient's mind is dissolved into its elements it then quietly waits until somebody puts it together again." This readjustment is an important factor in the process of analysis. Freud looks to the future rather as developing the further activities of the psychoanalyst in assisting the patient towards this automatic cure in another way. Active therapy, the latest development of psycho-analytic technique, is applicable when the improvement in the patient's condition hangs fire. This may take place when the patient is unable to overcome his fears and resistances, as for example in certain phobias. The physician must then use his influence to force the patient to face certain of these fears by making him undertake some part of the activity for which he has a phobia. For example, when a patient fears to go out, he must be made to do so, and as a result it is found that the nature of the resistances is disclosed and the analysis can proceed. Again when the patient has got so far better and reached a condition of comparative comfort it may be found that there is a delay in further progress, probably due to the fact that the patient is unwilling to give up the " advantage of illness " and face life without any " unconscious excuse." Under these circumstances it may be the duty of the analyst to " make things uncomfortable for the patient " by various prohibitions or commands related to positive or negative inclinations of the latter, so that he may acquire a renewed incentive to proceed with the treatment and effect a complete cure. Care must of course be taken not to com-plicate the transference by the establishment of too great antagonism.

Let us now consider the foregoing presentation *seriatim.* Few who have given serious study to the behaviour of neurotics and the genesis of their symptoms will be disposed to deny that these essentially depend on emotional conflict, repression, maladjustments of instinctive tendencies, regressions and the like, and therefore these need not be discussed again here. We are more concerned with the method of discovering and readjusting these difficulties within the personality. It must be understood quite clearly that psychoanalysis is a severe and often painful discipline for the patient and therefore should only be used for the more severe cases. There are many mild cases of neurosis depending on slight and temporary maladjustments in which it would be as absurd to apply psychoanalysis, as it would be to cut down and fix plates on a simple greenstick fracture of the radius in a healthy child. It must be admitted, however, that it is by no means easy always to be certain which cases will turn out to be simple and which complex, when they are first met with. Freud quite admits this and states that when the time comes for the treatment of many cases of neurosis in clinics, suggestion and hypnosis will once again come into vogue. For severe cases we must have some means of investigation into the unconscious impulses and conflicting emotional attitudes of our patients, and for this purpose some sort of psychoanalytic technique is necessary. Catharsis with abreaction, the revival of forgotten incidents with the " freeing of pent-up emotion " is successful up to a point, but, as Freud soon found, more was needed, and free association and the investigation of dreams would seem to be quite justifiable and likely to lead to useful results, but the process is long and the results confusing and the unravelling of the tangle must be left entirely to the patient. Even the technical improvements of concentration on the resistances and on transference rather than on forgotten experiences do not help much, and hence came the necessity for the classification of symbols. Here came the danger of going very badly astray. Admittedly, much in dream and neurotic material is symbolic, but it does not follow that what is a symbol of something for one person is necessarily a symbol of the same thing for another. Even the evidence of symbols having the same meaning in folklore and among primitives is not altogether convincing, for Rivers has shown that many of Freud's conclusions as to the meaning of primitive symbolizations and customs are superficial and inaccurate.[1] It is impossible to read the psychoanalytic literature on symbols without feeling that the writers start with a conviction that all the units of imagery which go to make up a dream or a myth must have a symbolic sexual meaning, and proceed to prove to their own satisfaction that it is so. Experience with patients, however, frequently seems to disprove this, both from their associations and from the therapeutic test, if this is of any value. The standardization of symbols then is apt to provide premises in a logical system, which may lead the observer lamentably astray. This wandering from the path of probability is often seen in those analysts who accept everything which is laid down by the master as an *ex cathedra* utterance. Their implicit belief seems to be due to a feeling of inferiority and a persecutory complex, which in spite of their confidence are exhibited all too frequently in the face of criticism. The same applies to the tendency to find universally applicable resistances, so that every female neurotic is jealous of her mother and every male afraid of his father and for this reason is suffering from his neurotic illness. In the same way " complexes " are standardized, and the Œdipus complex, the castration complex, and so on, are found in every case. I think there is little doubt that if anyone is subjected to psychoanalysis and the symbolism of their dreams and transference translated in the terms of the standard psychoanalytic glossary, some indication of one or more of these complexes will always be obtained, but to argue from this, that they necessarily are the roots of all neurotic illness may quite well be illusory, and personally I believe it is so.

[1] W. H. R. Rivers, *Psychology and Ethnology* (Int. Lib. of Psychol.). London and New York 1926.

The question of active therapy concerns us less here, since its value is not absolutely determined within the ranks of psychoanalysts themselves, but there does seem to be a full justification in making the patient face up to the necessity of the completion of his cure, and if by making things unpleasant for him experience proves that this can be done, it would seem a desirable modification of treatment.

A word may be said here on the view of psychoanalysts as to the relationship of their method to suggestion.[1]

Thus Ernest Jones [2] formulates three processes in suggestion : (1) *Rapport* between physician and patient ; (2) Inhibition of all mental processes except those suggested ; (3) The free development of the latter. The most important of these is the *rapport*, and for psychoanalysts this consists largely in the infantile attitude of the subject towards the operator, this being more important than the " power of the operator " over the subject. In both hetero-suggestion and auto-suggestion the subject regresses to a narcissistic level. In the former the operator is identified with the self, in the latter this identification is of course unnecessary. This regression is accompanied by the revival in the belief in the omnipotence of thought which is characteristic of the narcissistic stage. Without going further into the theory of narcissism here, the point is that from the psychoanalytic point of view, the two methods are diametrically opposed, and suggestion forces the patient back into an extremely infantile attitude towards the world, whereas psychoanalysis frees him from these infantile repressions and leads him to an adult state. That there is something in this is borne out by the fact that patients who have been treated by suggestive and persuasive methods sometimes do develop a dependence on their physician which is very hard to break.

[1] Cf. *Brit. Journal of Psychol. Med. Sect.*, III, p. 198.
[2] E. Jones, *Treatment of the Neuroses*. London 1920.

None the less for milder cases at any rate clinical experience does show successful results, without this too great dependence, and, as has already been said, Freud himself admits that these methods must be used when large numbers of patients present themselves for treatment.

The schools of Adler and Jung do not differ so much in the methods they employ as in the interpretations which they put upon their findings. Adler's defection from the psycho-analytic school was attributed by Freud to his own will to power which coloured the whole of his system of " Individual Psychology." The explanation of the neurosis according to this viewpoint has already been dealt with in Chapter IV and need not be repeated here. His method takes little account of repression and unconscious material, and consists more of an explanation to the patient of his line of life. He has sought to reach by circuitous means the desired goal of complete development and superiority, which has seemed unattainable, owing to his feeling of inferiority. These circuitous routes involve and employ the symptoms of illness which are used to establish superiority over the family and the environment. If we accuse psychoanalysis of being too systematized, this criticism is still more pertinent in the case of individual psychology, for every form of neurosis, if not all character-ology, is said to be founded on the masculine protest, on feelings of inferiority and compensatory will to power. That this theory throws a valuable light on certain cases of neurosis is unquestionable, but it certainly does not explain every case.

Jung's defection from the psychoanalytic school occurred soon after that of Adler, and was put down by Freud to a fear of the implications of sexualizing ethics and religion to which their investigations were leading them. Be that as it may, Jung's difference of methods depends on a difference in the methods of interpreting memories and dreams.

These are represented as depending not on sexual impulses, but on the impulses of life striving out to a higher ethical plane, and their sexual connotation, if present, is merely symbolic and not actual. He believes that what is obvious and conscious in the personality is compensated for by its opposite in unconscious life, and that these impulses will try to find expression through dreams and symptoms, and that the latter may be interpreted as an indication of the present and future tendencies in the patient's adaptation to life. The salient features of Jung's analytic psychology have already been dealt with, and it is only necessary here to point out its limitations. It is an essentially prospective system, and, as Freud aptly points out, tends if brought to its logical conclusion to become a didactic exhortation in ethics, which may be of the greatest service if the patient is sufficiently adapted to benefit by it, but in the case of the severe neurotic is often too difficult to follow, either intellectually or in his conduct. Again we must welcome the work of the Zürich school as a useful contribution both to psychological knowledge and to our armamentarium of therapeutics, but cannot admit it as a system of universal application.

If we may now summarize the conclusions as to the scope and limitations of psychoanalysis we may tabulate them as follows :

(1) It is necessary to select the case of neurosis which may be suitable for psychoanalysis, only the more severe cases showing a pronounced failure of adaptation towards life being suitable. It may only be possible to determine that a case is seriously maladapted, when the removal of a comparatively trivial symptom by some means clearly fails to cure the patient, but to the experienced physician the cases which mislead him in this way will become rarer and rarer.

(2) In these more severe cases, exploration of the conscious

S

memories and the removal of symptoms by suggestive means are not sufficient to cure the disease.

(3) Exploration of repressed memories, emotional attitudes to life and resistances are necessary to effect a cure, and for this purpose the only two possible methods are revival of memories with abreaction under hypnosis or in the waking state, and analysis.

(4) The former method is effective in the intellectual revival of images, but this is unimportant compared to the investigation of emotional attitudes and resistances; for the latter purposes, analysis is the only method.

(5) The methods of analysis are justifiable so long as the interpretations of the physician are not forced on the patient. The avoidance of this is very apt to lead to confusion of material and therefore short cuts are desirable.

(6) It is in the standardization of these short cuts, the typifying of symbols, resistances and complexes that danger lies.

(7) This danger is intensified in psychoanalysis since it is rigidly insisted that these are all sexual. This intensification of the danger of error is not necessarily due to their sexuality, but because this sets still more rigid bounds to the system.

(8) In the hands of wise and experienced analysts, there is probably little danger even from this systematization of interpretations, though it is noticeable that the system of the Freudians and that of the Adlerians and the Jungians are quite different and yet all claim good results. This is because in every case, in spite of academic differences, the good physician knows intuitively what his patient needs, and gives it him by one method or another.

(9) In the hands of unwise and inexperienced practitioners

the insistence on the rigid systems is dangerous, since they are apt to build false hypotheses on erroneous premises, and establish these as the basis of conduct and attitude towards life for their patients, sometimes with disastrous results.

(10) The practice of analysis is still a young art and must be left to develop or wither according as good results are established or not, but meanwhile much has been done by the movement to stimulate psychological thought, and for that we ought to be grateful. At present it ought to be regarded in the same way as is brain surgery for example. This is universally admitted to be a highly technical art and one which should be left in the hands of trained experts. The same applies to analysis.

(11) The idea that the medical treatment of the sick in mind can be safely left to those without knowledge of medicine, biology and psychology is absurd and pernicious, and has been responsible for much harm, as well as unjust criticism and abuse of the more orthodox practice, which should be regarded with watchful reserve by the intelligent medical and lay public.

One thing ought to be insisted upon in respect of analysis, and that is that its therapeutic effectiveness does not depend on mere intellectual enlightenment of the patient in respect of his past, but on the emotional adjustment which may be brought about by this enlightenment. Many people seem to be influenced by the ideo-motor fallacy. An idea can do nothing unless it acts as a stimulus to an emotional disposition. Any effective analytical treatment must therefore bring about an emotional readjustment of the patient towards life.

CHAPTER XV

THE SCOPE AND LIMITATIONS OF SUGGESTION IN TREATMENT

SUGGESTION has already been discussed at some length in connexion with hysteria, particularly in relation to the incidence of symptoms. It remains to consider it as a therapeutic agent. A great deal has been made recently of the supposed difference between hetero-suggestion and auto-suggestion, but the importance attached to this distinction seems to indicate a misconception of the nature of suggestion and the manner of its action. So far we have accepted McDougall's definition that " Suggestion is a process of communication resulting in the acceptance with conviction of the communicated proposition in the absence of logically adequate grounds for its acceptance," but before going further this requires some elaboration. Firstly, acceptance with conviction would be better expressed as—acceptance without opposition, which is not quite saying the same thing in different words. Acceptance with conviction seems to imply special facilitation for the pattern established, while acceptance without opposition implies an absence of inhibitions. Facilitation is more than a mere absence of inhibition, and the very nature and scope of suggestion does not imply any such positive effect as facilitation seems to be. In therapeutics the suggestive influence is generally an idea, and if we credit this idea with the positive influence of facilitation, we may easily slip into the error of the ideo-motor theory, which McDougall himself has done so much to explode, showing that it is the instincts or emotional dispositions and not ideas which are dynamic. What seems to happen is that the idea merely acts as a stimulus which starts the activation of a pattern involving affective-conative subpatterns, *i.e.*, emotional dispositions or instincts, and, so long as this is not inhibited by other patterns " set " in a contrary direction, the original pattern will continue to dominate the personality and determine behaviour. The stimulus may be a situation, a word, an image, a sensation or even an affect, and all these must be included in McDougall's somewhat narrow term " proposition," though this seems also to include the result of the suggestion as well as the source. If then we regard this as the way in which suggestion works, namely by setting off some already determined pattern, it is clear that the stimulus may arise either from the environment, in which case the process is called hetero-suggestion, or from the activation of another pattern in the patient's own ego, in which case the process is termed auto-suggestion. Hence there is no such essential difference between the two processes and they can be discussed together. Nor do we need to concern ourselves about the disputes as to whether M. Coué's methods involved hetero-suggestion or auto-suggestion ; they worked by suggestion and that is sufficient. The important point to remember is that we must avoid the error that is fostered by most popular writers on the subject, that the " implanted idea " can do anything. At the utmost all an idea can do is to act as a stimulus of activation to a pattern already existent in the patient's mental equipment, and if this activation is to be effective so far as behaviour is concerned, this pattern must not be seriously inhibited by contrary patterns. This conception explains a good many points in connexion with suggestion, its therapeutic effects and methods of induction. It is a truism that a subject cannot be made to do anything which is really against his will by suggestion. Under certain circumstances he will be made to do something which he does not positively wish to do, as in the case of post-hypnotic suggestions, such as commands to get up and shut the door in ten minutes' time. Such a suggestion may succeed because this pattern may have been activated and there is no definite contrary pattern inhibiting the action; but the subject cannot be made to murder his grandmother, because there are definite contrary patterns which inhibit such an action. Similarly suggestion is successful in removing neurotic symptoms when there are no definite contrary patterns to inhibit the recovery from these, but when a symptom is of real use to a patient in protecting him against some impossible, or very difficult demand in adjustment to life, or where a severe conflict exists between two patterns of almost equal consequence, then suggestion cannot achieve its object. It follows, therefore, that when the hindrance to adaptation is slight, the circumstances under which suggestion is given may make it possible for the more desirable pattern to become dominant, and a cure may be effected in such milder cases of neurosis. On the other hand, where the hindrance to adaptation is severe and deep-seated then suggestion is not effective, at least until some sort of analytic treatment has freed such severely afflicted patients from their resistances.

If the writings and recommendations of the practitioners in suggestion are examined, there is found a universal consensus of opinion that the patient must not exert his will, that he must be in a state of relaxation in which he is not attending to anything. The exertion of the will, so called, is a process in which at least the majority of the patterns making up a personality is integrated as an emergent whole in respect of an object or situation, and the rest of the patterns which constitute the personality are inhibited. Similarly, giving attention to an object requires at least a temporary constellation or grouping of emotional dispositions in relation to that object. These processes involve the functioning of the highest cortical levels, and it is clear that suggestion can only take effect when these functions are in abeyance, when one pattern involving cortical levels does not inhibit another pattern involving cortical levels, and when these patterns are in a state of loose combination, rather than in one of close integration.

As a therapeutic agent, suggestion is given when the patient is in a drowsy, hypnoidal or hypnotic state. The hypnoidal state is the condition between sleeping and waking, when the patient is still conscious of his surroundings but in which everything is in a state of poor integration and control. The hypnotic state corresponds, or is identical with the condition of sleep in which all cortical function is inhibited, as Adie, following the researches of Pawlow, has pointed out.[1] One is here postulating the possibility both of cancelling out on a vertical plane, if one may be permitted a spatial analogy, when patterns involving cortical and subcortical function are cancelled by each other's activities, and inhibition on a horizontal plane, such as occurs in sleep, when all activity at a higher level is inhibited from controlling and influencing activity at a lower level.

Sometimes distinction is made between two forms of hypnosis, one in which the operator commands and the other in which he persuades. This is really of very little importance, since some operators are more effective with commands and others with persuasion, while some subjects are more amenable to persuasion and others to commands. After all it is simply a matter of effective stimuli and attuned patterns, and these patterns will involve various emotional dispositions, such as self-abasement, sympathy, and the like. The depth of hypnosis is a matter of the degree to which cortical function, that is to say integration, discrimination and control are in abeyance. On the whole, therapeutic effects are most likely to be favour-

[1] W. J. Adie, *Brain*, III, 1926.

able when hypnosis is light, because then there is more chance that the patterns affected by the stimulus of the suggestion will be rearranged and integrated as part of the whole personality. On the other hand, if the hypnosis is deep, there is so much temporary dissociation of the personality, that while any isolated pattern may be set into activity by the stimulus of the suggestion, and so more or less bizarre or remarkable behaviour may be induced and scraps of memory be revived, such behaviour and images are less likely to be permanent once the patient is wakened from hypnosis, since the activated pattern has not had a chance to be integrated into the personality as a whole.

M. Coué's methods were undoubtedly successful in certain cases, but his explanations or rather those of his apologists, like Mr Harry Brooks,[1] were anything but convincing, and too sweeping assertions were made as to their efficiency. Probably the chief value of his teaching was to induce his patients to relax and cease to pay attention, so that the suggestions of his formulæ were enabled to achieve success. The success however was limited to relatively mild cases, in which there was no marked inhibition to recovery of health and no deep-seated conflict which could only be resolved with difficulty.

To tabulate the scope and limitations of suggestion as a method of treatment we may say :

(1) Suggestion acts as a stimulus to patterns already laid down in the personality.

(2) Such patterns may become dominant and may determine behaviour temporarily or permanently, provided there is no serious resistance from other patterns.

(3) Suggestion will be most effective when the integration and mutual resistance of patterns is partially relaxed, in such

[1] H. Brooks, *The Practice of Auto-suggestion.* London 1925.

a way that the activated pattern may modify the personality more or less permanently. Under these conditions neurotic symptoms may be permanently removed.

(4) When the integration is too much disorganized, as in deep hypnosis, marked effects may be produced and old memories may be revived, but these may only be active while the state of deep hypnosis is still present, and when the patient wakes, the symptom which has been removed is apt to reappear, and the memory which was revived carries no conviction as being part of the personality. Hence the therapeutic effect is less valuable.

(5) Suggestion involves a *rapport* between operator and subject in order that the stimulus may activate the pattern.

(6) In auto-suggestion this *rapport* is organized within the self-regarding sentiment, but may induce a regression to an introspective (narcissistic) attitude.

(7) In hetero-suggestion there is a danger that the subject may regress to a state of dependence on the operator, unless the relationship involved in *rapport* is recognized and too great dependence guarded against.

(8) Suggestion is a quick, useful method of cure in mild cases of neurosis, when there is no serious opposition to recovery and no deep-seated conflict.

CHAPTER XVI

THE SCOPE AND LIMITATIONS OF PERSUASION

CONSIDERABLE interest was aroused before the war, by the methods of Professor Dubois of Berne [1] in his treatment of neurotics. A clear-minded, upright and persuasive individual, he tried to treat these patients by exhorting them to more sensible and rational behaviour. Owing to his own personality he achieved considerable success, but his methods have not obtained similar results in other hands, which shows that a good deal of this therapeutic method depended on suggestion. Déjérine [2] adopted a similar method, but recognized the importance of emotion in the genesis of the neuroses, and tried to work out a method of combining the persuasive rational treatment of Dubois with the investigation and explanation of emotional reaction which Janet [3] practised, but the result was rather confusing and has not led us very much further. These methods are applicable in cases in which the maladjustment to life is a perfectly conscious one or when, if the patient is not conscious of what is wrong, he is perfectly capable of grasping it, directly it is pointed out to him. It is specially applicable to certain mild cases of hysteria, those referred to in Chapter VIII, which depend on a definite suggestion either from the organic illness of the patient himself or from some obvious external agencies such as have been described. Two errors seem to exist in respect of this " persuasive " treatment. In the first

[1] Dubois, *Les Psychonévroses et leur Traitement Moral*. Berne 1908.
[2] Déjérine and Gauckler, *Les Manifestations fonctionelles des Psycho-névroses, leur Traitement par la Psychothérapie*. Paris 1911
[3] P. Janet, *Principles of Psychotherapy*. London 1925

place, those who practise and pin their faith to it are apt to expect that all cases of neurosis should yield to it, and think that if they do not, the patients must either be perverse and unwilling to get well, or else of weak intellect, so that they cannot grasp the explanations which are given them. This is of course quite unjust to the patient, who is suffering from more severe forms of neurosis. For example, if a patient is suffering from severe anxiety, it is no use to ask him why he has this unpleasant symptom or to exhort him not to have it. He has not the least idea as to why he has anxiety, what it means or has relation to, and since it is there and he would give everything he has not to have it, it is not of much use to exhort him not to suffer from it. Again, if a patient has a phobia for a dark room, we may exhort him by telling him to pluck up his courage and assure him that there is nothing to be afraid of in the dark room, and we may even persuade him to enter it, but he will not do it naturally and easily, until it is discovered by some analytic method what he is really frightened of, for the dark room is only a symbol of the real trouble.

On the other hand those who habitually use analytic methods are forced to admit that a certain type of patient is cured by these persuasive methods, but they are inclined to deny that such should be included amongst the neuroses. Of course it is easy enough to say that neurosis depends on repressed conflict and that anything which does not do so is not neurosis, but if the conditions which are included here are not neurosis, what are they? They fit into a progressive scale and it would be difficult to determine a point when this ' X ' disease passed into neurosis. To deny these milder conditions inclusion amongst the neuroses is rather like insisting that tuberculous infection of the lungs is only present when there are definite signs of cavity formation and hæmoptosis. For example, consider the boy troubled over the problem of masturbation and suffering from quite marked anxiety because he has acquired this habit, which he finds hard to give up, and because he fears that if he persists in it the most dire results will ensue. He knows exactly what is the matter, but he needs help, and unless he receives help he is not only ill at the time, but is in a fair way to repress the whole business later and develop as severe a neurosis as the most enthusiastic psychoanalyst would wish to tackle or to avoid tackling. Not only does such a problem become complicated by accretions with the passage of time, but regressions occur and difficulties and conflicts of earlier childhood become involved in the complex whole. Again with the milder hysterical symptoms, as has been shown, they may or may not be involved in a pattern which is part of a neurotic complex, and, if they are so involved, then this other manifestation must be dealt with as well as the hysterical symptom, but if not, the latter may be dealt with by itself and for itself. It was of course during the war that the hysterical symptom which was susceptible to cure by persuasion alone was most common, and those of us who worked at Seale Hayne realized how much could be done by this method.[1] There is of course no doubt that our enthusiasm carried us too far, and we believed that we had cured many cases which afterwards relapsed and had to be treated by more elaborate methods, and that we did not always recognize the underlying mental condition, which urgently required help, but the fact remains that we did cure a great many patients who did not relapse, since, with the removal of their symptoms, their adaptation to life again became normal. Such cases are certainly not nearly so common in civil life, since self-preservation in war meant disability, while self-preservation in peace generally means physical fitness. Hence symptoms are not in harmony with this important pattern during peace-time, while in war-time, they were

[1] *Seale Hayne Neurological Studies.* London 1918.

easily associated with this. None the less they do occur, and no medical officer in charge of a physiotherapy department of any hospital, who is on the look-out for these cases, is long without seeing one who requires treatment. The method of dealing with such a case is to investigate the origin of the disability and explain this to the patient, so that he understands why his disability has arisen and what is its nature. This is specially necessary since without it the patient cannot give up his symptom without loss of self-respect. Then he is told to perform the function which is in abeyance, for example to move his leg, and encouraged to make a real effort. The result is much more likely to be successful if the function can be restored completely at one sitting. This was possible when we were whole-time military officers, doing all our work in one place, and when it did not matter if we gave up even several hours at a stretch to one patient, but it is not easy to do this under the conditions of a hospital out-patient department, though it may be managed by arrangement in private practice.

It is often necessary to carry on a certain amount of re-education in order to restore proper postural tone in long-standing cases. The normal postural or resting length of muscles alters if the limb is kept for long in an abnormal position, and until this normal condition is restored, movements take place at a disadvantage ; moreover the patient should be encouraged to use the restored function as soon as possible, preferably in some useful and interesting occupation. To sum up the scope and limitations of persuasion we may say :

(1) Persuasion alone is quite useless in the cure of the more complicated cases of neurosis.

(2) In those fairly numerous cases in which the causes of maladaptation to life are definitely known by the patient, or which can be easily grasped when explained, persuasion may be remarkably effective.

(3) In the removal of hysterical symptoms which are simply the habit continuations of previous suggestive effects, persuasion is the method of choice.

(4) The good effects of persuasion depend largely on the enthusiasm, confidence and personality of the physician and the extent to which these appeal to the patient, for the same physician, however skilled, will not be equally effective with all his patients.[1]

---

[1] With reference to the last three chapters we may compare McDougall's *Apologia pro psychotherapeutica sua*, to which I am most certainly willing to subscribe.

" I believe in the value of mental exploration as deep as the case requires ; and I regard free association and dream-analysis as important methods of exploration. But I also hold that exploration in hypnosis is in many cases useful and entirely justifiable. I believe that conflicts and repression are principal factors in the genesis of functional disorders ; but I believe that emotional shock or trauma also plays a great part in many cases. I believe that sexual difficulties are one of the great sources of disorder ; and that early sexual strivings and repressions may in some cases prepare the way for later disorder. I am even prepared to admit that sexual stirrings may occur in infancy in an uncertain number of persons and that in all probability, such persons are peculiarly liable to neurotic disorder in later life. But I believe that functional disorder may and often does arise independently of the sex instinct. I do not believe that the Œdipus complex is formed in all infants and is the main root of all neuroses, dreams, religion, morals and civilization in general. Nor do I believe that the symptoms and other expressions of repressed and dissociated systems are determined in form by a cunning, designing activity which seeks to render possible a partial expression in disguised form, in order that the ' Unconscious ' (or any part of the personality) may enjoy the pleasure or satisfaction of such expressions."

" Readjustment is, I think, the best term for the designation of the second great stage of the psychotherapeutic process. (The first stage is that of exploration.) In many cases something may be done by modification of the environment, especially in the case of young people, where the errors of well-meaning parents play so large a rôle in the creation of conflicts ; but all such modification lies outside the actual scene of the psychotherapeutic process. The most desirable procedure, possible only with patients of good intelligence, is to help the patient to understand the genesis of the disorder, to lead him to a critical evaluation of all the factors involved and, where necessary, a revaluation of them and to inspire him to the adoption of a new attitude dominated by some strong purpose ; to set before him some worth-while goal towards which he may strive, sustained by motives which he wholly accepts and approves, and which are in harmony with the whole of his character. In all this there is much scope for intellectual activity ; the patient may achieve a revaluation of various factors by considering them upon a broader background ; and he may achieve a more single-hearted, dominant purpose, or a more harmonious system of dominant purposes, by facing and thinking out more thoroughly than he has previously done his own nature, situation, and problems.

" The mere adoption by the patient of a detached, objective, critical, intellectual attitude towards his affects and emotional problems tends powerfully to render him less the sport of his impulses, takes something of the tang and poignancy out of his emotion, renders him more master and less slave, of his affects. In all this the physician may play a useful part of a kind that may be regarded as purely intellectual, by putting before the patient wider and wiser points of view. But this work cannot be separated from the moral influence of the physician ; and if the physician is in satisfactory rapport with the patient his influence may be very great in leading the patient to adopt the wider and wiser standpoint, to make a better evaluation of factors, to adopt satisfactory purposes, to aim at worthwhile goals from satisfactory and harmonious motives. In all this if the patient respects, admires, and trusts the physician, the latter inevitably uses the power of suggestion, whether unwittingly or intentionally ; and it may fairly be supposed that, other things being the same, the physician who uses suggestion deliberately but tactfully, with clear understanding of what he is doing, will use it more effectively than he who uses it unwittingly and at the same time indignantly denies any imputation of resorting to such an ' inferior ' procedure. It should not be forgotten that suggestion may be used to induce belief in what is true, even more effectively than to induce belief in what is false."—W. McDougall, *Outline of Abnormal Psychology*, pp. 480, 470. London 1926.

CHAPTER XVII

THE PATIENT AND THE PUBLIC

In concluding this discussion of the Neurotic Personality, it seems worth while to refer to the relation of the patient to the public at large and the attitude of the man in the street to the neurotic.

Unquestionably the neurotic is frightened of the public, for he feels that people do not understand him, that they think he is a malingerer or a degenerate, and that they may have knowledge of some guilty secret which he scarcely dare admit even to himself.

Sometimes the hysteric seems to be an exception to this, for he appears almost to flaunt his disability in the public eye, but if a close watch is kept, it is found that this flaunting is rather in the spirit of " a poor thing but mine own," and he does it to buttress his own failing faith in the efficacy of the physical substitute for mental distress.

One of the greatest difficulties which the neurotic has to face is his sense of isolation. Practically every patient believes that no one has ever behaved or suffered as he has done, and this is chiefly because the public makes no effort to understand him. Another difficulty is that the neurotic does not understand himself, and so it comes as a surprise to him that the physician does try to understand him and even succeeds in doing so. It is often found that the first establishment of a satisfactory transference dates from the time the physician tells the patient what he is feeling before the latter has related his own troubles. Moreover these troubles seem nonsensical to the patient, and he is so used to being told that his complaints are all nonsense and if he would only buck up he would be all right that he is unprepared to find anyone taking him seriously. If it was not pathetic it would be tedious to listen to the constantly reiterated statements : " Oh, of course you won't believe this "—" You can have no idea what I go through "—" No one knows how I suffer," and so on. He is told so often that his symptoms are imaginary, that they are not real, that he begins to wonder whether such a unanimous opinion must not be right, and yet he knows that he tries, that he struggles against his symptoms, and so he is further mystified and frightened. Moreover he is dimly conscious that his neurosis depends on a guilty secret, and this incidentally is actually the case, and he is terrified that it is somehow displayed in his face or his manner, so that all the world knows what he does not clearly know himself. In relation to masturbation fears, this is explicable when one considers the frequency of " bogey " threats, such as the statement that the spots of acne so common in adolescents are directly caused by masturbation. Pernicious lies like this are implicitly believed by large portions of the public and may be the source of untold torture to the neurotic.

The next question which arises is why the public so persistently misunderstands and refuses to sympathize with this class of patient. The attitude is one of almost studied cruelty, and in the vast majority of cases cruelty depends on ignorance and fear. The tendency to be cruel to things we fear and cannot understand is illustrated all through history in the persecution of new ideas and bizarre discoveries. The public as a whole is ready to pour out any amount of sentimental sympathy when the patient has anything to show, but when the patient merely complains of vague and illogical fears and uncomfortable but quite incomprehensible sensations in his inside,

T

people have no time for him, they cannot see and do not understand what is happening, so they dismiss it as impossible.

Another factor is of great importance in determining the attitude of the public. As has been said, every one is a potential neurotic and given a sufficiently difficult situation to face, he would break down under the strain, and every one has a horrible half-formed fear that in looking at the neurotic he ought to ward off the evil eye and murmur : " There, but for the grace of God, go I." There is always something fearsome and uncanny in the caricature of oneself, and this is what the neurotic is, though perhaps few may admit this, until they have studied the neurotic reactions and recognized their almost logical inevitability, given the requisite premises. When we have studied these, it appears as if the public wilfully mis-understood the neurotic, but that is because people take the neurotic symptom at its face value. They cannot understand why a person who is not nervous of, say, flying in an aeroplane, should have a nervous breakdown, and show all the signs of anxiety or terror when there is apparently nothing to provoke this. The nervousness or the lack of nervousness in flying depends on the nature of the sentiment in relation to passenger flights. In every one the emotions grouped in relation to this object will include fear, self-assertion and curiosity. The two latter condition each other to constitute a sense of adven-ture, and if these are strong enough to become dominant in the sentiment, fear does not intrude unduly, because the whole sentiment is organized at the level of consciousness, where discrimination and control are possible, and the patient knows exactly what he is afraid of and how much he is afraid. Under such circumstances he goes on his flight and enjoys it. On the other hand if fear dominates in the sentiment, again he knows exactly what is happening and he stays on the ground. Sup-pose, however, that at first our subject manages to fly reason-

ably comfortably, till one day the aeroplane has to make a
forced landing, then fear is enormously intensified and
becomes dominant, so that the balance within the sentiment
is changed and he permanently or temporarily loses his
nerve for flying. Under ordinary circumstances this is taken
philosophically, and he merely says to himself, " I never knew
flying could be like that, and now that I do know, I am
jolly well never going to fly again." He makes no secret of it
and does not feel embarrassment about it. But suppose that
flying was his job or had assumed some symbolic significance
for his personality, such as the ideal pursuit for a courageous
man, such as he wished and believed himself to be. Then if
he finds himself frightened of flying he loses his self-respect,
there is a conflict ; he does not come up to his ideal of himself,
and a similar situation arises as that which pertained in the
war neurosis, so that a real nervous breakdown may ensue.
However, the alarming experience in the aeroplane is only
the trigger which fired the gun, so to speak, and the neurosis
depends on and is kept up by the endopsychic conflict in
relation to the self-esteem. Thus we see that while, under
special circumstances, losing one's nerve for something may
be the starting-point of the neurosis, it can never fully explain
it, and in the vast majority of cases has nothing to do with
the real neurosis and represents a totally different process.
Similarly with other etiological factors, so dear to the public
mind, such as overwork, influenza, and the like, they may,
by reducing the powers of adaptation, allow conflicts for which
a compromise had been found to become so insistent that
the compromise no longer suffices and neurosis results. For
all that, they in no way explain the neurosis and their elimina-
tion by no means necessarily cures the illness. Further,
the apparently illogical anxiety is a symptom of conflict
and is not the same as a fear of definite objects.

It was a matter of great mystery to many people that the

declaration of the Armistice did not immediately cure all war neuroses ; as a matter of fact it cured scarcely any and intensified many, though eventually it did much to make cure possible. The public however regarded war neurosis as pure funk of war conditions, oblivious of the fact that unrestrained fear could no more cause neurosis than unrestrained courage. There must always be conflict and the emotional opponents of fear of war comprised in the ideal of self were as much injured by the Armistice as fear was relieved, for there was no longer a chance of making good and so rehabilitating the patient in his own regard. Similarly, in the peace-time cases, removal of the obstacle to one side of the conflict does not always clear up the situation, since the other side cannot adapt itself to this removal.

If the patient can come through to the other side of neurosis he is generally the better man for it, since he has a greater understanding of himself and a wider comprehension of the difficulties of others, and if the public were made up of cured neurotics, the patient would not have such a bad time and would certainly get better more quickly.

Life is growing faster and more complicated, and more and more people fall by the way and fail to achieve adaptation to rapidly changing circumstances. Must we wait then until all the world has had a breakdown, before we can look for justice to and understanding of our neurotic patient ? I think not. If we can spread an understanding of neurosis and abolish the fear of it, we need not condemn every one to undergo the experience in his own person.

First of all the public must be taught that the neurotic is a really sick man, that he is undergoing serious suffering and is deserving of much sympathy.

Secondly, it must be learnt that this suffering is the result of a perfectly definite cause, as definite as a broken leg or infection with the bacillus of influenza, and that therefore the sympathy must not be merely passive but must aim at putting the patient in the way of a cure.

Thirdly, that while cure must depend on a comprehensive view of the whole neurotic personality, it will be achieved rather by psychical than by physical means.

Fourthly, both the patient and the public ought to be protected from the seductive but misleading advertisements of quack nostrums, which at best act by suggestion and at worst poison the patient. These frequently neutralize each other, since each and every friend and acquaintance the patient meets has his own pet panacea which he fervently recommends. Usually the patient tries one after another for a time, and then consigns the whole lot to the devil and the sink, and no great physical harm is done, but valuable time is lost and confidence of the patient in any sort of cure is seriously undermined.

Fifthly, the public ought to learn that once a patient has undertaken a course of treatment on any reputable line he should be allowed to continue along that line for a reasonable time free from counter suggestions of better treatments to be obtained elsewhere.

Sixthly, it must be realized that the neurotic is not insane, and that he is not going to be a danger to himself or other people. As has been said already, it is often very difficult to distinguish between early cases of certain forms of insanity and neurosis, and mistakes in diagnosis go far to mystify and confuse the public mind on this point, but increasing knowledge and experience on the part of doctors ought before long to make this a diminishing difficulty.

Lastly, the public must understand that by endeavouring to appreciate the difficulties and sufferings of neurotics and to understand the way in which they are brought about, they are achieving more insight into their own personalities and thereby diminishing the chances of breakdown in their own persons.

Such a flood of literature on the subject of the neurotic

and his treatment has appeared of recent years and so many people have put forward their views as to how he should be dealt with, that both the public and the patient are apt to lose their way in the labyrinth. The cynic may argue that when so much is written, little can be known, and the unfortunate patient is apt to think that he is but a plaything tossed about amongst practitioners, who are still groping in the dark and who seek him to provide them with experimental material whereby they may peradventure find a little light. To my mind, however, such opinions are ill-founded, for the confusion is more apparent than real. Since every neurotic is ill because he has failed to adapt himself to some situation either within his own ego or in his environment, he must always present a different problem from that of his neighbour. Further, it by no means follows that there is only one possible path whereby he may seek and find readaptation. Not only will a physician choose different paths for his various patients, but it is also possible that a patient might be guided along different paths by different physicians with equal ultimate success. The shortest and most satisfactory path in any individual case must depend, not on any stereotyped rule of treatment, but on the adjustment and relationship between the personalities of the patient and the physician he chooses. For this reason it is no wonder that the literature abounds with so many manuals of treatment which are dissimilar and even contradictory, and all of which may yet be perfectly correct under the circumstances in which the treatment is given. It is on these grounds that I have striven to survey the possible methods of treatment rather than lay down any hard and fast lines on which this should be carried out, for I believe that any given line of treatment must be inapplicable in a large percentage of cases, and what the physician requires is the judgment to know what particular form of treatment will help his patient most. Furthermore,

I believe that although the last word has not been said on neurosis, sufficient is known of the subject to enable us to assert that every case can be helped and that a large majority can, to all intents and purposes, be cured by one method or another. It behoves both the patient and the public to recognize that neurosis is an illness, that it is an illness due to a failure of adaptation, and that the patient cannot find adaptation by himself without the greatest difficulty, that the longer the state of maladaptation persists the more complex does the illness become and the more difficult and tedious the cure. Treatment should therefore be sought early and not late, and it should be understood that though it will be conducted chiefly by mental means and not by means of the orthodox bottle of medicine, there is nothing in this which pertains to the magician or the charlatan, for everything is connected in a perfectly logical scheme.

INDEX